CROOKED
Man-made disease explained

The incredible story of metal, microbes, and medicine—hidden within our faces.

by Forrest Maready

FEELS
LIKE
FIRE!

All rights reserved. Published in the United States by Feels Like Fire, an imprint of Feels Like Fire.

ISBN 978-1983816628

Printed in the United States of America

Thank you to my wife & research partner, LeAnne.
This book would not have been possible without your indomitable
spirit, your inquisitive mind, and your constant support.

There is the unknown and there is the unknowable.
We were made to figure out the difference.

A NOTE FROM THE AUTHOR

A few years ago when I first started noticing people had crooked faces, I could not have imagined the chase it would lead me on. It started as a simple search for what was causing our lopsided smiles and misaligned eyes, but over the next two years, it would transform and focus every waking (and sometimes sleeping) hour of my existence into an attempt to understand if crooked faces might actually be a common thread that tied all of the "modern" diseases together.

Who am I to suppose I could discern the answers to riddles that have been vexing the world's physicians and scientists for two hundred years or more? I am not a scientist. I am not a physician. I am no one, not even a hobbit from the Shire. I studied music and religion in school, playing the compositions of Bach on the pipe organ and dissecting the works of Gerard Manley Hopkins. I excelled at neither.

But my mind was on fire—always. A cosmic game of connect-the-dots spinning in my head, latching on to the most trivial details from an important lecture while forgetting all that was significant, storing them in my brain for later retrieval in an organizational system that made no sense. I was always learning—just the wrong things at the wrong time.

Eventually, after having acquired enough wrong things and after having connected enough dots, a pattern emerged—a curious constellation that was both intriguing and horrifying. It became clear to me much of the sickness and suffering that currently plagues humanity was man-made—all due to an entirely noble attempt to help each other with a decidedly ignoble result.

This book—this story, represents the journey I undertook, the connections I began to see, and the theories (or *hypotheses* as some of my actual science friends will insist they be called) describing how our bodies are not only being harmed, but more importantly—how they might be healed.

The ideas presented in this book are theories, or hypotheses, if you will. They have come from a very comprehensive study of medical history and the most recent scientific research available. I may speak with confidence within as if I am sure of everything I say. Without the encumbrance of putting a giant disclaimer on every page, realize that *I do not know* if these things are true. I believe them to be true. Indeed, I am terrified they may be true. But it is important that they be discussed, mulled over, researched and either tossed in the trash or acknowledged. If my theories are wrong, I can go back to looking for a nice hobbit-hole in which to smoke my pipe. If they are right, well then perhaps there is more hope for healing and recovery than any of us thought possible. Perhaps we are ready to depart this age of man-made disease after all.

INTRODUCTION

In all of human history—the pocks and pustules, the fevers and fatigue, the nausea and neuropathy—every symptom of disease we have ever experienced is the result of the body trying to rid itself of a perceived invader. Even the fatigue and ensuing sleep that often went along with being sick were specifically requested by the body in such a way as to maximize a response. Whether the intruder was a trivial invader or posed a genuine threat to life, disease was the necessary side effect of healing.

It may seem that today is no different than two hundred years ago, which was no different than two thousand or two million years ago. It may appear that all of the effects of disease we see today are simply the body recognizing an invader and trying to either kill or expel it. Whether the attack be viral or bacterial, our body may give the appearance it is responding to the assault the exact same way today it did thousands of years ago.

What if all of the modern diseases that have appeared in the last two centuries actually follow a different pattern? What if something unique happened recently that in the previous millions of years of history had never happened before?

As it turns out, something *did* happen. Something *did* change that I believe will one day divide the whole of human history in two. Humans began digging ore from the earth's crust and extracting the metals contained inside—a process that would help create the biggest leap in industrial, agricultural and technological progress the world is likely to ever see.

But that is not the demarcation. During this period, humans began to ingest and inhale these metals. At first, accidentally—through the lead water pipes of 3rd and 4th century BC Mesopotamia or the mining of the materials themselves. Later, the metals would be found to have some medicinal value, and humans began to ingest them—purposefully. Their danger became well known, but with the knowledge of the human body and disease so primitive, the extent of damage the metals were doing was woefully underestimated.

The era of "metallic medicine" truly began in the late 1700s, when old ideas about how to treat sickness experienced a revival and led to frequent prescriptions of mercury and arsenic containing pills, tonics and powders. The next 100 years of human civilization would be a horrible chapter in the history of medical care, as the treatments used during this period undoubtedly killed far more people than they saved.

Despite this suffering, toxicity from heavy metals was muted until the late 1800s due to the methods by which they were administered—through ingestion. Because they were taken orally, most of the heavy metals were blocked by the intestines and excreted before they caused much harm. This might destroy one's teeth and bowels in the process, but it achieved the desired effect—to purge whatever might be ailing the body (along with everything else in the intestines).

If it seemed ineffective at curing the ailment, dosing of the mercuric medicines might be increased until "salivation was achieved."

Inevitably, enough of the metal would be absorbed into the body from whence a thousand different maladies might spring forth. It's little wonder the 1800s is known less for its medical miracles and more for its asylums and fainting rooms.

In the late 1800s, the toxicity of metals would exponentially increase. The syringe, having recently gained popularity with morphine injections, was to create a more direct pathway into the body. While the intestines were an efficient barrier, the rest of the body was not. Injections bypassed all of the sophisticated protection of the gut and gave metals free entry directly into the vulnerable organs inside. Even the kidneys and their miraculous abilities of filtration struggled to excrete tiny amounts of injected metal.

Before this time, the body's immune system had only organic matter to deal with.[i] Its white blood cells could enclose and destroy any microbe it encountered. Metals present a unique series of challenges the body does not have an answer for. White blood cells cannot destroy it, so the metal will exist as a toxin inside the body until it is converted into another form or excreted—both of which might happen over a period of years, even decades, rather than hours or days.

Probably the cruelest aspect of these medicinal metals was recognized two hundred years ago, something authors of that era might refer to as a "Vicious Circle." Metals hijack the immune system itself in such a way that your body's natural response to harm creates more harm. Which creates another immune response, which metals use to create more injury. And on and on it goes—a process which might explain why such tiny amounts of injected metal seem capable of causing so much damage.

Unfortunately, the era of metal is trending towards another century of human suffering and heartache. There are over 100 autoimmune disorders, many of which did not exist until recently. There are many

---

i. Allow me this gross oversimplification for now.

new pediatric and geriatric neurological illnesses that make the misery of smallpox and polio seem trivial in comparison.

The suffering of humanity due to ingested, inhaled, and more recently injected metals, may one day be remembered as one of the cruelest periods in modern history. The fact that these metals were administered—often against the desires of parents and their children, and at the behest of public health officials and their legislative enablers —does little to lessen the heartache.

But a thorough understanding of what may be causing our afflictions should bring more hope than sadness. The guilt which may come with the realization that what we're experiencing is partly our own doing will be difficult. However, the likelihood we will be the generation to end this scourge upon our species should cast more light than a thousand suns upon our despair.

With this optimism, I hope that you will read through this book and begin to acknowledge where we went wrong. I believe that with the understanding of the nature of man-made disease, healing will be an inevitable consequence. And finally, I pray that all of those who have suffered or died from the mistakes of this terrible period will not have been in vain.

METAL & MEDICINE

"In natural action, there is a consent and symmetry in every part."

— *Charles Bell, The Anatomy and Philosophy of Expression*

This section focuses on the beginning of man-made disease which started in the early 1800s when metals began being used as medicine. It also looks at the many parallels between modern illnesses and disorders that started appearing at that time.

A FLICKER OF LIGHT

It was for me, the first of a few seemingly unconnected observations. A flicker of light out of the side of my eye. A small door appeared where before, there had been none.

A family friend called me one morning in obvious emotional distress. There had been trouble rousing his son from sleep that morning and they had rushed him to the ER. Eventually, little Joshua had come to, but it was clear he was having profound neurological trauma. Seizures. A dagger through any parent's heart. Hospital staff were having trouble getting them under control. A helicopter flew them to a bigger hospital with more specialists. More seizures. More questions.

What had happened? Joshua had seemed perfectly fine, his smile and gregarious personality beamed rays of joy everywhere he went. Not a sign of anything wrong. Like everyone that knew the family, we sat by our phones, checking emails, messages, anything for a sign of hope that the boy would be okay. It sounded bad. Survival was all we prayed for.

* * *

A few months later, I found myself looking through Joshua's family blog for any signs as to what might have gone wrong. Scrolling through each post, I was reminded of how healthy and vivacious he had been. Picture after picture of a smiling, happy boy. His parents, doting on him, as any parent would, enjoying each and every milestone. As the posts got closer to the date of his seizures, I analyzed everything. Each event, each picture, looking for any clue as to what might have caused his sudden illness.

The last post before he was airlifted to a regional children's hospital caught my eye. Joshua sat on the floor, a toy in his hand, looking playfully at the camera. But his face looked different. Something was off. His mother had noticed it too. The picture was captioned "Don't you love his cute crooked smile?"

Once I noticed it, it was obvious. His face drew up on one side into a smile. The lip turned up, his cheek puffed out and his eye "squinched" with happiness. But the other side of his face did nothing. His lip turned very little, and his cheek was flat, which gave the eye above it a rounded appearance. One side of his face looked happy, but the other side did not. I went backwards a few posts and found another nearly identical picture of him—but this one was symmetrical. In fact, as I combed back in time through every image of him I could find, I never saw his face looking different. It was always straight. Yet here was this one picture, two days before he would need to be airlifted in a frantic attempt to save his life. It was vaguely similar to the media campaigns teaching how to spot the symptoms of an impending stroke in the elderly. But this was Joshua. He had just turned 18 months old, and his face was sagging on one side. Just like the posters.

Perhaps it was a flash of light, a clue I should have reacted more strongly to. Regardless, I didn't think about it again for several months. The seizures were under control and less severe, but it was clear that Joshua and his parents had an epic battle ahead of them. Joshua was lucky in one important regard—his parents were ready.

Months later, I was going through some older photo albums my mother-in-law had dropped off at our house. There were two books, both of them dedicated to the first 20 years of my wife's life. School pictures, sports pictures, Christmas time and playing at the beach. The square pictures with the rounded corners glued underneath the plastic film lack the detail of any modern photograph but somehow provide clarity the new ones cannot.

As I thumbed through the first album into the second, my wife joined me, providing back story for each shot.

"Softball team," she said, pointing at a tiny girl standing in the back row with long brown ponytails underneath her red baseball cap. "I was the fastest runner on the team."

I rolled my eyes as I flipped into her high school era photographs.

"Was," she said, for clarification.

I stopped at a large yearbook picture, taken when she was sixteen years old. She had transformed, in the turn of a few pages, from cute softball-playing tomboy into a beautiful, young woman. I had seen a smaller version of the photo before—it was one of my favorites of her.

"Look at my smile," she said to me as she stopped me from turning the page.

"What is it?" I asked her.

"Look at it," she said again as she put her finger on the page. "It's crooked. Look how it turns down on the side."

I never consciously thought about it before, but now that she pointed it out, I saw it. In fact, I think it was one of the reasons that picture had been my favorite. A sly, cheeky smile that belied an innocent-looking girl who knew far more than she let on.

"It wasn't always that way," she said, as I turned backwards and started looking through the previous pictures for similarities.

Again, a small flash of light. Barely enough to register, but it was there, tickling my brain.

"When did you get sick?" I asked her out of curiosity. I knew it had been sometime in high school—fatigue, weight loss, Crohn's disease. The older pictures, going back in time, were all looking symmetrical.

"It would have been around Spring 1995. I got my wisdom teeth out at Christmastime, got a massive infection that wouldn't respond to any antibiotics, and within a few months…"

I pulled the picture out of the album, looking for a timestamp on the back like the old pictures had. "That would have been your Junior year, right?"

"Yes, and that's my Junior year photo. I know it already."

A year later, I got a cryptic message from an old friend of mine I hadn't spoken to in years. Robert knew I had been the subject of a documentary on Discovery Health Channel about my especially picky eating habits and was curious if I might know anything about his particular issue. He was concerned about his hearing.

"I have issues with processing sound," he wrote, "specifically in differentiating between important sounds and background noise."

After having spent years in the film industry working in audio engineering and sound design, I was intrigued.

"To clarify," he continued, "I expend a great deal of energy in trying to listen to and understand what someone is saying, for example, because I am unable to filter out other voices, atmospheric noise, background music, etc."

"Have you had your hearing tested?" I asked.

"I literally hear everything," he said, bluntly.

I knew of something called hyperacusis, though I didn't know much about it. It was a common sensory issue in children with autism —what I remembered as an increased sensitivity to sound and often the reason you see children with autism wearing earmuffs when out in public. I asked about any neurological issues and he jokingly confirmed he had been able to overcome his ADD diagnosis with "over-caffeination."

On a whim, I asked Robert if he could send me a picture of himself when he was younger. His mother was a photographer, and as a result he had a very clear picture of his infant self, sitting in a high chair.

I immediately noticed his mouth, perhaps even his jaw, drooping to one side. But he was in a high chair, probably eating something. Baby's mouths do weird things when they eat.

"Do you have a later picture of you, preferably smiling?" I asked.

He went through his yearbook, grabbed a grainy black and white picture of himself and sent it to me.

It was instantly obvious. Robert's smile was crooked. One side worked, the other didn't. Even more pronounced than Joshua's or my wife's. His lopsided mouth from the baby picture may have been due to him eating, but based on the high school picture I was looking at, I guessed not.

I sat back in my chair, my hands pressed to the side of my head. The light no longer flashed—it streaked across my brain, bouncing around the inside like a thousand tiny ping-pong balls. It was clear to me, something was happening to our faces. But I had a vague feeling… more unease than anything—it wasn't just our faces.

EVERYWHERE & NOWHERE

After the exchange with my friend Robert about his hearing, I began to notice these crooked smiles everywhere. What I had previously attributed to a smirk, I could now see was actually a facial palsy—muscles on one side of their face were not working properly. Sometimes it was dramatic, other times more subtle.

The internet provided an unlimited source of photographs, and Hollywood answered the call with thousands upon thousands of pictures of people smiling. As I began scanning through red carpet and publicity photos, I noticed the crooked smile everywhere. There were a few smirks here and there, but I thought surely not everyone in Hollywood smirked at every photo opportunity.

Two curious patterns began to emerge as I logged hundreds of pictures with crooked smiles. The first: it was mostly males. I noticed a few females with asymmetrical smiles, but in general there were very few women with crooked smiles. The second pattern was more odd: Most everyone's smiles, when crooked, were higher on the right side, lower on the left. It seemed this pattern was just as distinct as the gender difference. Every now and then you would spot someone smiling with the left side high, right side low, but it was remarkable how often the opposite occurred: when they tried to smile, the left side of their face would not do what was asked of it.

I knew that males got autism more often than females, but with our understanding of ASD and its origins so spotty, I couldn't make a connection. However, the tendency for left side paralysis over the right was absolutely confounding—it made absolutely no sense to me. The only lateral distinction I could think of within the whole of humanity was left or right sided preference with writing, throwing, or kicking. Between 70% to 90% of humans prefer to use their right side for most tasks,[1] and I recalled a foggy notion that one side of the brain controlled the opposite side of the body.

Neither of these peculiar patterns made any sense to me, so I filed them away in the back of my brain alongside many other questions that had begun to emerge.

Another facial anomaly began to surface as I looked through thousands of photographs. It wasn't just our smiles, but our eyes. Something was off. Many people, although I wouldn't describe them as cross-eyed, had something noticeably different. One of their eyes might have turned the slightest bit outwards, while others would have an eye that was turned in. The outward turned eye was very subtle for most people, but when their eye turned inward, it was hard to miss—it felt like something might be wrong. Like the smiles, once I noticed the crooked eyes, I began to see them everywhere, cataloging the misalignment among celebrities, athletes, news reporters, doctors. I would freeze frame commercials on TV, take pictures of realtors on billboards and rip pages out of magazines. It seemed like no one was immune from this phenomenon.

I began to question whether humans had always looked like this.

People's faces couldn't be completely symmetrical—I remembered some web pages where they would feature the image of a famous celebrity with a little slider you could drag from side to side, mirroring either the left or right halves of their face. It was often comical how different someone could look if their face was perfectly symmetrical.

In an effort to maintain my sanity, I started researching some of the oldest images of photography. Daguerreotypes exploded into popularity in the 1840s, when painted portraits were an impossibility for most. Until that time, paintings, drawings and death masks were about the only way to capture the likeness of someone. Daguerreotypes provided an incredible amount of detail, the likes of a which a painted portrait would never capture, and at a cost much cheaper than hiring a painter for hours, possibly days, to paint your family portrait.

In the 1840s, Daguerreotype photographers began to advertise in newspapers and walk along busy thoroughfares, touting their new technology. Collections of these old images revealed a common subject —family portraits featuring a recently deceased child, dressed and posed amongst the living as if nothing were wrong.

As I poured through image after image of these early photographs, I rarely, if ever, was able to spot anyone's eyes looking anywhere but perfectly straight ahead. It was remarkable how perfectly aligned people's eyes appeared during this time period. It also became obvious there was never a crooked smile because quite simply, there was never a smile at all. The instantaneous click you hear on your phone that now simulates the opening and closing of a camera shutter used to take as long as five minutes—for a single image. The daguerreotype process had a major flaw in that it was not very sensitive to light and needed to be exposed to the subject matter for minutes rather than milliseconds.

These extended exposure times were the impetus behind the "hidden mother" photographs, where you see a child held tightly in place by a figure completely obscured by a blanket, tablecloth or curtain. It also created the need for posing chairs, curiously designed furniture that hid a small, padded headrest behind the portrait subject so they could more easily hold a steady pose. Portraits taken under these conditions were grueling, as one had to remain perfectly still for extended periods of time. It's not difficult to imagine how holding a smile for five minutes would be painful, so everyone in these early photos adopted neutral facial expressions that required little effort to maintain.

Photographic technology progressed into the 1860s and 1870s and as exposure times improved, a few daring souls began to experiment with more relaxed poses. These photographs took a little work to find, but over a few weeks I began to assemble them from various collections around the internet, always notable for their rarity—someone from the 1800s, smiling.

As creepy as the post-mortem and hidden mother photographs are, the rare glimpses of humans smiling almost one-hundred and fifty years ago are a complete joy. Like the older daguerreotype images I had looked at previously, everyone's eyes seemed aligned perfectly. But unlike the older studio portraits, their locations were more varied: An older couple at a wedding party. A group of boys, clowning around on top of a fence. A mother and daughter, posing for a portrait in the garden outside their house. Several young children, now without the hidden mothers required to hold them in place. And all of them were smiling. Perfectly even, level smiles. Both cheeks puffed out, both eyes squinching evenly with happiness. It was remarkable.

During my research, I was occasionally able to find someone with a misaligned eye. They were extremely rare, but there was a haunting image of someone from an insane asylum who's left eye had turned so far outward it was only half visible. There was a civil war soldier whose eye turned in severely. After looking through hundreds of images, I only saw a few misaligned eyes. Besides a very odd-looking Edgar Allan Poe, I never spotted a truly lopsided grin like you might instantly find today by searching the web for "crooked smile."

It was apparent to me that humans had not always looked like this, at least not in the severity or ubiquity that existed today. I thought perhaps only the most photogenic of humans decided to be photographed, given that it was still a relatively expensive undertaking. So I looked through a large collection of mugshots from Australia in the 1920s. These characters looked to be straight out of a Hollywood central casting agency—gangsters, thieves and prostitutes with tussled hair, scared faces and broken noses, but again, the symmetry was remarkable. You could look through a hundred or so images before you spotted one person with asymmetry.

"Confirmation bias theatre," I kept telling myself. I had caught a whiff of a peculiar phenomenon, had a hunch it was a relatively recent occurrence, and in a human-powered search for answers, had constructed the perfect set of images to fit the narrative I wanted. It was classic confirmation bias. There was no way these crooked faces could have only recently come into existence.

As it turned out, I was right. Asymmetrical faces had previously existed, and in the early 1800s, an inquisitive physician from Scotland was determined to understand why.[2]

CHARLES BELL

Charles Bell had an inauspicious start to his career. At the beginning of the 19th century, surgeons were known not so much for their stethoscopes and scrubs as they were their lancets and *scarificators*—disturbing-looking implements used for purposefully bleeding patients in a somewhat misguided attempt to heal them. Bloodletting had been a common medical practice for hundreds of years, and as other young surgeons beginning their training had done, Charles Bell vomited violently upon his first attempt at the practice.[3] He would eventually move on to what many would find even more stomach-churning—studying anatomy and neurology.

Like many physicians of his day, Bell became proficient in creating detailed illustrations of the anatomy he studied. There exists a famous painting which depicts a man deep within the throes of a tetanus infection, his body arched high up into the air, fists clenched in pain—that is a painting done by Bell.

As he expanded his anatomical knowledge, Bell dissected the most intricate webs of nervous tissue that seemingly branched and forked at random and was amazed at the realization they followed the same exact pattern he had seen in other patients. It were as if he'd found a beautiful tree in London, mapped it down to the tiniest branch and twig, travelled to Paris and found the exact same tree. A sense of awe and religious wonder permeate the documentation of his discoveries. While veins and arteries could differ wildly, the nervous system followed a distinct set of instructions so specific as to defy belief.[4]

One of Bells' contributions to medicine was a much clearer understanding of how the nervous system functioned, something that was poorly understood at the time. He recognized there were two types of nerves—ones that controlled movement—*motor nerves*—and others used for sensing things—*sensory nerves*. He also realized there were special nerves which could apparently serve both motor and sensory functions simultaneously.[5] Fortunately for Bell, experimentation on animals didn't have the stigma of today, so by severing the various nerves of dogs or monkeys and observing the often horrible effects, he was able to build a composite of which fibers controlled and sensed different areas.

The cranial nerves, then still an enigmatic bundle of twelve fibers emanating from deep within the brain, drew most of Bell's attention. These nerves emerge from the brainstem and snake their way around inside the head, through holes in the skull and into the nose, the eyes, the tongue, the ears and other places. They are numbered in the order in which they surface on the brainstem, front to back. The 10th, commonly referred to as the Vagus nerve, was especially peculiar as it connected the brain to everything from the mouth and esophagus to the heart and intestines. Bell was consumed with understanding the 5th and 7th seventh cranial nerves which made up the sensory and motor nerves that controlled and sensed the face.[i]

Some of the facial palsy that Bell observed could be attributed to physical trauma. Like the animals he experimented on, a fractured skull or enlarged tumor could sever or damage one of the nerves controlling the muscles in the face. The areas of the face these nerves controlled would sag and the muscles themselves would waste away from lack of use. Sometimes their forehead could wrinkle on one side yet remain completely smooth on the other, an effect they found very odd. Liquids would run out of their mouth when they tried to drink. They would need to manually close an eyelid with their hand, sometimes taping them shut so they could sleep comfortably.

This disorder had implications beyond vanity as Christians of that era were fascinated with one's *countenance*—how one's facial expressions and emotions reflected the depth of their spiritual faith. Fields of study related to this effect were plentiful—anthropometry, phrenology and physiognomy, to name a few. These overlapping disciplines employed intricate mappings of facial features and skeletal measurements to determine and predict anything from someone's intellect to their likelihood of committing a crime. Racial overtones were always present, as were lofty descriptions and drawings of one's own phenotype. Bell was no exception to this craze and spent page after page dissecting the divine countenance clearly observable within the European face.

Because of this, many people were deeply troubled to find something so visibly wrong with their visage. It was even more disturbing when facial palsy began to appear minus obvious physical trauma. For many, there was no kick to the head from a horse, no horn from an ox or fall from atop an apple tree. Their faces had become

---

i. In medical and scientific literature, you will see them referred to with Roman numerals—cranial nerve V and cranial nerve VII. Because Roman numerals are slightly outmoded, this book will make use of Arabic numerals.

paralyzed, and no one understood the reason. Facial palsy had been clearly mentioned as early as the 9th century by a Persian physician,[6] but during the 1820s, Bell gave a series of presentations to the Royal Society in London documenting something very new. Many of them were cases of facial paralysis he had been made aware of by colleagues. Others were patients he had treated himself. His familiarity with the details of partial facial palsy and treatment led physicians to refer to this phenomenon as Bell's Palsy.

Unfortunately, it is nearly two hundred years after the formal declaration of this disorder and we usually don't know why it happens. It often follows a specific viral infection, such as Herpes Simplex or Epstein-Barr, the virus that causes mononucleosis. It often occurs during pregnancy, for reasons unknown. Some suggest the viral infections can get into the cranial nerves, causing paralysis. On their circuitous journey from brain stem to their final destination, cranial nerve fibers pass through tiny holes in the skull called *foramen*, creating vulnerable "pinch-points." Because of this, some have theorized swelling from the infection may cut off the blood supply, causing miniature strokes within these susceptible sections of the nerves.

If you conduct research on Bell's Palsy, you will notice scientific articles state the cause of Bell's Palsy as *idiopathic*—unknown. They will also state that Bell's Palsy is the most common cause of facial paralysis.[7] It doesn't take a physician to realize this medical sleight-of-hand presents the patient with an impotent diagnosis that essentially means "We don't know why this happened."

Bell's Palsy is a terrifying disorder that fortunately will often resolve on its own after a few weeks, sometimes months. Scientists don't know why it happens, but I was beginning to think that understanding the mechanism for facial paralysis might explain a lot of things.

BABIES

At this point, I had seen hundreds of pictures of people with crooked smiles. It seemed to be everywhere. But I had been looking through celebrity photos, not normal people. Not kids, and not babies.

"Was this something you just pick up as you get older?" I asked myself. "Could this be an inevitable consequence of aging?"

I opened my laptop and did a search for "crooked smile baby." I was shocked to see them everywhere. Some had the characteristic lopsided smile—what might be called a smirk. Others featured one side of their bottom lip looking completely paralyzed, so much that it drooped down and to the side. I cataloged these images, looking for other patterns: gender, race, hair color, etc. It was a large collection of crooked smiles, but none of them had a backstory that might provide more clues.

I widened my search and began to look through many of the parenting forums that intrepid mothers use to ask each other questions, often when they were unable to get satisfactory answers from their pediatricians. The tone of the posts ranged across the spectrum of emotion.

"Anyone else have a little guy with a crooked smile?" a mother asked. "Look how cute he is. Show us your crooked smile babies!"

Whether she was actually worried or not, I couldn't tell, but she was at least seeking some kind of reassurance that her baby's face was normal. A few other moms responded with pictures of their own. Some voiced concern. Another mom posted a picture of her son with the foreboding subject "Neurologist appointment."

"Little man had his one-year old checkup today," she wrote. "The first thing the pediatrician said was how happy he was and he had big sweet smiles. Then she said his smile was a little crooked and put in a referral to see a neurologist. I am so worried, so upset, so sad, been crying my eyes out all day."

It doesn't take reading many posts like this to realize the tightrope pediatricians must walk every day when they spot what might be a problem. They want to communicate concern to the parents, but know that any tiny blip on the radar may be perceived as possibly life-threatening.

The mom attempted to reassure herself. "My little guy is perfect just the way he is and his smile totally melts my heart. His smile and laugh are what makes my day. I honestly never noticed it being crooked and now I'm so upset to think something could possibly be wrong. I just don't understand."

Given the apparent ubiquity of crooked smiles, this pediatrician might be commended for saying something. Yet still, if you are a parent, you can sympathize with this mother. The bolt of fear a doctor can strike through your body with just a few words is terrifying.

Another mother submitted a picture of her son for analysis to a new-mothers forum. "I've noticed that my little one's mouth leans to one side when he smiles. I haven't noticed it when he cries, only when he laughs/smiles widely. It's kinda freaking me out. Has anyone ever seen or experienced something similar? Should I be worried? I just didn't know if it meant something could be really wrong? Because it's never gotten better and reading about it has me all sorts of stressed my dear son didn't have this when he was born."

A third mom wrote of recent experiences with her son. This one mentioned other things which I would later become particularly concerned with.

"Little one has always had a symmetrical smile. But about 4 months ago all the sudden he has this crooked or half smile. Anybody else dealt with something like this? The change in his smile also started about the same time he started blinking a lot and randomly shutting his eyes real tight. Other than these things he's completely happy and healthy and on track with milestones. Should I be worried??"

Like any of the other posts in this vein, I wanted to reach out to these mothers and ask them if everything was okay. I wanted to know what had happened to their precious children—little boys and girls that had begun to display what in the past would have seemed like a trivial change in their face. Now, I had begun to develop the same concern these parents had. Was this crooked face just another freckle? Nothing to be concerned with? Or was it a warning sign that somewhere within their cranial nerves—or possibly deeper within the brain stem itself—something was going terribly wrong?

STRABISMUS

I'll never forget the first time I spotted something wrong with a child in real life. It was a beautiful little black girl who was sitting on the counter at the bank next to me. She was probably four years old, facing out towards what must have been her grandmother. Her hair had been styled into little pony tails, fastened together with the same colorful, plastic-ball hair ties many of my classmates from elementary school had. I couldn't help but to glance at her. She was unwrapping a lollipop the teller had given her and sensed I was looking. Without moving her head, which was pointed directly forward, she looked up at me. Actually, one of her eyes looked up at me. The other did not. It moved to the side, but just barely.

I caught my breath as she looked back towards her grandmother. Her eyes had snapped back into perfect alignment—nothing apparently wrong. But from where I was, when she looked up at me, it was obvious —one of her eye muscles wasn't working properly. I looked at her grandmother, oblivious to my unease. She would have never seen it, never spotted it, had she not been in the exact scenario I just witnessed:

her granddaughter, without moving her head, looked up and to the right. It was strabismus, a dysfunction of one of the six muscles that control the eye. And more concerning to me—it was glaring one moment, and gone the next.

Humans, like many other predatory mammals have both of our eyes facing forwards. This arrangement favors depth perception over an increased field of view. Many animals of prey, like rabbits or antelopes, have eyes on the side of their head. This provides them a wide field of view, allowing them to see far behind without having to turn their head. When your eyes face in the same direction, you can only see a narrow field directly in front of you, but gain a distinct advantage—something called binocular vision. With binocular vision—with two eyes in slightly different positions but pointing in the same exact direction—your brain can sum these two images together into one picture, yet triangulate the differences between them to determine how near or far away something is. It's a remarkable computation, a trigonometric miracle that happens hundreds, possibly thousands of times a second without you even being aware of it.

For prey, distance calculations are unimportant. Any predator is danger, near or far, and being able to spot them before being spotted is paramount. For predatory animals, correctly judging the distance of your prey as you quietly stalk upon them, as close as possible, could mean the difference between your survival or death from starvation.

As a newborn baby grows, they develop two separate systems that allow them to see—sight and vision. Sight is the perception of light upon the retina in the back of your eye, which is converted into neuronal signals and sent to the brain via the 2nd cranial nerve, the Optic nerve. Vision is what allows your brain to take these two separate images and stitch them into one coherent picture of the world in front of you. Other parts of your brain then kick in to interpret that image—

What is close? What is far? What is red? What is green? What is safety? What is danger?

A remarkable component of human vision is facial recognition. Infants seem to display an marked interest in human faces before nearly anything else. Indeed, babies as little as two days old appear to mimic human expression.[8] Our vision seems remarkably tuned to recognize and store the subtle distinctions between millions of faces, and a story my father relayed to me would confirm this.

He had just turned eighty years old when he walked into the lobby of a restaurant and was greeted enthusiastically by an older man seated by the door.

"I know you," the man told my father as he tried to stand up and shake his hand.

"I know you," my father replied, vaguely recognizing him.

They began to cycle through their childhood histories, searching for where their paths might have crossed but were thrown off as the older man was ninety-four, nearly fourteen years older than my father.

"Comment vous appelez-vous?" the man asked, throwing back his head with laughter. "I taught you French."

Instantly, my father realized who the man was. It was his French teacher, from high school. The older man, unsurprisingly could not remember my father's name, but out of the thousands of students he had taught, and out of the millions of faces he had seen over the years, he had instantly, nearly sixty-three years later, recognized my father, now looking much different than at seventeen-years old. The facial recognition capabilities of the brain, along with its ability to store these unique patterns and account for the drastic changes faces undergo over decades of aging is nothing short of astonishing.

Once someone has developed both vision and sight, abrupt changes to any of the components in this process can create problems—one of which is *strabismus,* a condition in which one or more of the muscles that control the directional movement of the eyes don't work properly.

This can sometimes result in an obvious impairment noticeable by an eye that is turned inwards or outwards. It can be less obvious, sometimes completely hidden or only apparent when the eyes are turned towards an extreme range of motion. The functioning eye will move where the brain wants it to go, but an eye with muscle weakness will sometimes not aim correctly.

If you research strabismus, you may see it pop up under the term "squint." There are parts of the world, such as India, that still refer to it this way. Squint originally referred to a condition relating to the eyes that was caused by the 7th cranial nerve, the facial nerve. Part of the function of the 7th cranial nerve is to enervate the muscles that extend and retract your eyelids. When a particular part of this nerve develops problems, you might have trouble fully retracting your eyelids. You may have actually noticed this in someone and never realized it—this condition often gives the appearance of looking sleepy despite them being well rested.

If your eyelids are not retracting properly, it can also give the impression that you are squinting. As additional maladies around the eye began to be described, such as misalignment issues, they were often grouped under the umbrella term squint. Nowadays we have nomenclature for specific types of strabismus, but a few countries still refer to it by its original name: squint.

The eye has six different muscles that allow it to point in any direction. There are four muscles where you might expect—on the top, bottom and both sides. The other two wrap around and attach on the side of your eye furthest away from your nose.

The top and bottom muscles are controlled by the 3rd cranial nerve. They are what allow you to look up and down, and are the reason you rarely see strabismus where one person's eye deviates upward or downward. If you develop a problem with your 3rd cranial nerve, it may impair your ability to look up or down as far as you would like, but because they are working (or possibly *not* working) in tandem, both the top and bottom of the eye are likely to be equally weakened. The left and right sides of the eye are controlled by different cranial nerves. When both of these cranial nerves are working correctly, the eye is held perfectly in balance. If one of these cranial nerves develops a problem, the eye will often no longer be centered.

In addition to up and down movement, the 3rd cranial nerve is what pulls the eye inward, towards the nose. If you develop a problem with the 3rd cranial nerve, your ability to pull the eye inward will be weakened and your eye will tend to deviate outwards. This is called *exotropic strabismus*. If you develop a problem with your 6th cranial nerve, which normally pulls the eye outward, the 3rd cranial nerve on the inside of your eye will have more power and will turn your eye inward towards your nose. This is called *esotropic strabismus*.

Once your brain has developed vision and is combining the two images from your eyes properly, developing strabismus will cause vision problems. You will have double vision because your eyes are now pointing in different directions than they had previously and the vision part of your brain, which had trained for so long to combine the two images perfectly, is still combining them the way it was taught. But other parts of your brain recognize the problem—there are now two slightly offset images which don't merge into one the way they used to.

This problem can obviously affect reading, but even if your child is too young to read, it can affect their ability to play, eat, and even interact with others. A common solution is to prescribe special glasses called prism glasses. These glasses are not built to correct nearsightedness or farsightedness, but have tilted lenses that are designed to redirect images going into the eye at the original angle, an effect which should correct the double vision.

Perhaps all strabismus is not bad. An interesting pattern I have noticed is that exotropic strabismus, where an eye points outward, is remarkably common amongst athletes. So common, in fact, that I wonder if it doesn't present a distinct advantage in depth perception. I once cataloged images of the top four tennis players in the world at that time—Roger Federer, Rafael Nadal, Novak Djokovic, and Andy Murray and they all seemed to display a form of strabismus (amongst a few lopsided grins). Like the crooked smile, once you begin to notice eyes not lining up, you will see it everywhere.

I still wasn't convinced that crooked smiles and misaligned eyes had always been with us. In an effort to understand their prevalence— and perhaps their cause—I began to read through the accounts that Charles Bell had gathered. What I discovered was a remarkable pattern that consistently pointed to the same cause.

BELL'S FIRST TWO CASES

Between 1821 and 1829, Charles Bell presented six papers to the Royal Society in London covering his research and theories regarding human anatomy and the emerging study of the nervous system. Amidst his papers, he presented 89 different medical cases dealing with facial paralysis and other forms of the illness. A few accounts included multiple people with similar symptoms, and others were notable for the thoroughness in which their maladies had been documented.

Reading through these cases is both enlightening and horrifying. Enlightening, in that the stories and symptoms are varied and paint a broad picture as to the kinds of ailments people were suffering at the time. Horrifying, in that after reading these reports, one cannot escape the realization that both patient and doctor from today—with similar conditions—often appear as equally flummoxed as they were then, nearly two hundred years ago.

The first case was in the form of a letter submitted to Bell for examination. He presented it to the Society:

* * *

No. I

"It is in my power to relieve your mind of much anxiety. My experience has furnished me with five cases of paralysis of the muscles of the face of one side, completely local, and in no way connected with the encephalon[i]. They all did well without general bleeding. Dr. B. and Dr. S. met me lately in consultation on the case of a lady in the eighth month of her pregnancy, who suffered this partial paralysis of the muscles on one side of her face, from the action of mercury on her mouth. The sore mouth inflaming, a lymphatic gland between the mastoid process and the angle of the jaw compressed a branch of the seventh pair of nerves. The muscles of the face on that side were so completely paralyzed, that the cheek was drawn by their antagonists, and the mouth disfigured.

"Dr. B. and Dr. S. suspected pressure on the brain at the origin of the fifth pair of nerves. But I took the liberty of stating the discoveries of Mr. Charles Bell, and proved to them, by other cases which had fallen under my notice, that there was no danger, and that the brain was not implicated.

"This case, in the course of a fortnight, did well under the use of mild laxatives, leeches behind the ears, and a small blister."[9]

If you are new to the study of 1800s medicine, you will undoubtedly remark at the treatments administered to the pregnant woman in this case. Laxatives, leeches and a small blister may not seem customary, but a quick description of these treatments is in order. A small "blister" would have been created either with noxious powders or a hot iron applied to the skin, a technique that was still being recommended into the late 1800s as a treatment for infants who had been stricken with paralysis. Leeches would also have been applied in the same hope—

---

i. *The brain.*

drawing out the infection or toxins causing the problem.

Laxatives were a problem in and of themselves. The "mild" descriptor used in the testimony is a subjective term, as a popular remedy of the day, Dr. Rush's Bilious Pills, were also referred to as "Thunderbolts" or sometimes "thunder clappers." Whether or not thunder clappers were thought to be mild is up for debate, but we can be sure their main ingredient, mercury chloride, was not treating the patient gently. Most medical treatments of that era were centered around cleansing the bowels—purging, it was called. If the purgative didn't bring relief, dosing was increased until the mercury produced salivation—a sign which was evidently positively thought of. Regardless, if you had nearly any illness and went to see a doctor, you could be assured either the contents of your stomach were coming up, or the contents of your intestines were coming out. Sometimes both.

The doctor indicates the other patients with facial paralysis did well "without general bleeding," a procedure that was still popular amongst the most forward-thinking doctors at the time. Although bloodletting, blistering and purging were the go-to trinity for medical treatments of the day, the doctor specifically attributed her facial paralysis "from the action of mercury on her mouth." Another popular medicine of the day was simply called a "blue pill." Most didn't have a brand name associated with them as the local pharmacy would have compounded them according to whichever recipe they were fond of. Regardless of the specifics of the recipe, blue pills (or blue mass as you will sometimes see them called) would have at the very least contained a good amount of mercury chloride, if not pure elemental mercury.

Blue pills were used to treat everything from syphilis to tuberculosis. Although they were also used to ease the pains of childbirth, we can assume this poor lady was prescribed them to deal with constipation, a frequent occurrence during the later stages of pregnancy. The mercury pills had evidently made her mouth sore, a common occurrence with mercury poisoning, but her paralysis was attributed to a swollen lymph node—a result, no doubt, of the mercury —presumably compressing the blood supply to the cranial nerve controlling that side of her face.

Whether this diagnosis is correct we cannot say. Thankfully women are usually no longer prescribed mercury containing products,[ii] yet still, Bell's Palsy is more common during pregnancy. Tumors are known to occasionally cause cranial nerve palsies in this way, but as for lymph nodes swelling to such size and firmness as to preclude oxygen flow to the nerve—that is not a commonly observed phenomenon. Never the less, the treating doctor believed the facial palsy was due to the mercury pills she was taking and prescribed some minor bloodletting (via leeches), blistering and more laxatives—additional medicine that we can only assume contained more mercury. The blistering, laxatives and leeches seemed successful in treating the facial paralysis, but it was likely the cessation of blue pills that had the most effect.

Other cases would follow this seemingly comical pattern of treating medicine-induced sickness with more of the same. Another case is worth looking at:

> No. VII
> "Mary Unwin, now in the twenty-second year of her age, is about seven months advanced in her second pregnancy: she is of a full habit of body, and instead of having the usual wasting of the face and sharpness of features, she has a plumpness and fullness. She has for some time complained of spasms of the lower extremities. Her constipated state of bowels has required powerful purgatives to relieve her... She applied for advice respecting a remarkable affection of her face, on the 5th of February. On examining the countenance, a single distortion of

---

ii. As of early 2018, some forms of the flu shot still contain Thimerosal, a mercury compound. Old habits die hard.

*the features is most apparent. The mouth is drawn to the right
side, and the nose evidently inclines in the same direction… In
sleep, the right eye-lids are closed as usual, but the left eye
remains uncovered… There is occasionally a dimness of vision of
the left side..*"[10]

Another pregnant woman is presented with facial palsy on one side.
Interestingly, the doctor mentions that she was administered
"powerful" purgatives to relieve her constipation. Whether these were
more powerful than Dr. Rush's Thunderbolts we do not know, but as far
as I can tell the relative strength of purgatives was simply adjusted by
adding more or less mercury to the recipe. He mentions she
complained of "spasms of the lower extremities." Knowing that
mercury poisoning can cause muscle tremors[11] and twitching[12] should
make anyone realize the medicine she was receiving for constipation
was undoubtedly working in more ways than they imagined.

Later, she developed facial palsy on one side of her face. Her mouth
was drawn to the right side, because it was the side of her face that was
functioning correctly—the left side had developed palsy. He also
mentions an occasional dimness of vision on the left side, another
symptom of mercury poisoning.[13]

Here was another case of a pregnant woman who was administered
mercury-laden medicine and subsequently developed facial palsy. It is
impossible to determine if this woman's facial palsy was caused by
mercury, but as I began looking through Charles Bell's 89 cases of
paralysis, the administration of mercury containing medicine followed
by paralysis would become a common theme that was difficult to
ignore.

BELL'S THIRD CASE

The surgeon was developing the reputation of a capable physician, and consequently the scope of ailments with which he dealt began to grow beyond facial palsies. Mysterious new disorders   seemed to appear every day, but Bell, like other physicians, seemed intent on using these cases as a key to better understanding the nature of the human body. As to the source of their cause—that was a question no one appeared to be asking.

Bell had been able to recreate the facial palsy he had seen in patients by severing the 7th cranial nerve in animal models, but upon reading through some of the other case studies he presented, it became apparent that disorders of the 7th cranial nerves were just the tip of the iceberg. It wasn't just the face—the problems were everywhere.

No. IX

"Geo. Bungay, æt. 20,[i] was admitted under Dr. Macmichael's care, November 22d. He had symptoms of fever for a week before he presented himself at the hospital. He complained of getting no rest at night: his bowels were constipated; his tongue foul; the pulse slow and regular; he had slight tenderness in the epigastrium[ii] ... In the afternoon of the 25th he was seized with delirium; the delirium came on in paroxysms. After this he fell into a comatose state. He continued in this state until his death, which happened on the 29th... When the delirium came on, it was observed that the right eye remained always closed, while the left eye was opened: he had lost the power of raising the lid of the right eye. Upon elevating it with the finger, it was discovered that he had also lost all motion of the eye-ball: while the left eye revolved from one side to the other, this remained still, and as if he were looking straight forwards ... Dissection.— On raising the brain from the basis of the skull, both the optic nerves, but in particular the right one ... was found to be a thick deposit of coagulable lymph, straw-colored, and of the consistence of jelly ... it is to the coagulable lymph matting the third, fourth, fifth, and six nerves together, that you must look for an explanation of the symptoms in regard to the condition of the eye."[14]*

The sequence of events involving George Bungay's treatment will become familiar. He had symptoms of a fever—possibly a garden-variety sickness. Whether he had been administered medication for this fever or not is unclear, but the complaint of a "foul tongue" is a dead giveaway for mercury toxicity. There are some modern medications that can create a strange metallic taste in your mouth, but in the early 1800s, the only thing known to cause this would have been a metal or metalloid like mercury or arsenic.

---

i. *Around 20 years old.*
ii. *The part of the upper abdomen immediately over the stomach.*

In the hospital, his mention of "foul tongue" would have not set off any alarm bells for poisoning, so his complaints of constipation would have likely been addressed with mercury-laden purgatives. Three days later, this poor soul, already showing signs of mercury toxicity, began to suffer delirium—another indication of toxin issues.

During this period, he lost the ability to elevate his right eyelid—a sign of 7th cranial nerve palsy. The doctor discovered after manually retracting his eyelid, the eye had also lost all ability to move—a rare indication of both 3rd and 6th cranial nerve palsies, if not also the 4th.

George Bungay would die in the hospital, seven days after he was admitted. The physicians treating him would no doubt feel they had given him the best care available, but despite their best intentions, even a hasty review of the literature suggests they may have killed him quicker than nature could have. The same sequence of events that may have created a 7th cranial nerve palsy was also causing problems elsewhere—in the eyes.

It was clear to me the crooked smiles and misaligned eyes I was noticing everywhere wasn't a completely new phenomenon. Crooked faces, which in the past might have been attributable to a tumor or traumatic blow to the head, had begun to appear in greater numbers—around two hundred years ago—when physicians started aggressively using metals as purgatives for nearly every illness. Medicine was administered, then crooked faces would appear—a disturbing pattern that would unfortunately continue for a very long time.

MEDICINAL METALS

Ancient Romans had issues with lead poisoning, and even Chinese emperors from thousands of years ago apparently died from arsenic or mercury poisoning.[15] If these metals were known to be so toxic, and had been administered anyway for hundreds of years, one might ask why it became such a problem in the early 1800s?

The medical revival of an old theory began in the late 1700s, based on Hippocrates' concept of disease and sickness being related to the four humors—black bile, yellow bile, phlegm and blood—being out of balance. This renewal, starting in the 1780s, is referred to as the age of "Heroic" medicine. According to Heroic theory, the way to restore balance was through careful and copious (emphasis on copious) amounts of bloodletting, sweating and purging. Blood had been drained by the liter for thousands of years and sweat lodges had also existed since time eternal, but this era brought forth a renewed zeal for these practices that undoubtedly set the progress of medicine back a century or two.

Purging became an extremely popular remedy during this time and consequently doctors began prescribing mercury-based medicines for nearly anything. Even babies were not immune, as Dr. Stedman's Teething Powder ("Absolutely Safe and Harmless") became a popular treatment for infant teething pains. It was simply a pill in powder form and was not rubbed into the gums, but placed on the tongue, chased with a swig of milk and was intended to purge the poor child of anything that might be causing their imbalance.[i] Other mercuric medicines arrived on the scene in addition to some popular arsenic-based products. It would seem that opiates were the only medicine they were prescribing at the time that likely did not kill anyone—ironic considering this once popular medicine is illegal in many states today.

With a massive increase in the popularity of doctors prescribing medicinal metals to every man, woman and infant in Europe and the United States, we would expect to see a rash of new problems appear. Although they were aware of the dangers of mercury toxicity at the time, they didn't understand the mechanism by which it harmed.

Like other metals, mercury does most of its damage to the neurological, gastrointestinal and renal (kidney) systems. Elemental mercury—the silver compound in its raw form—was rarely used for medicinal purposes other than instrumentation. Although you often hear about it being accidentally ingested, it is most toxic if inhaled—the reason for which entire buildings are evacuated when someone breaks a thermometer. Calomel, the mercury often used in purgatives of the day, was poorly absorbed by the intestines but with the "heroic" doses that were being administered, it was enough.

Trauma to the head could sever a cranial nerve or a strategically placed tumor could cut off its blood supply. But something about the medicinal metals that were being administered *en masse* were also

---

i. Any lingering curiosity as to why "polio" was often referred to as "teething paralysis" by mothers in the early 1800s has faded due to the apparent success of the polio vaccines.

causing problems with cranial nerves. They were the source of other issues—muscle spasms, delirium, and death—but something specific was happening with metal and the cranial nerves, as if they had an affinity for one another.

Mercury can bind to the cells of any organ and prevent them from working. When enough cells are damaged, the organ itself will cease to function. It can also penetrate and damage a protective layer—called the blood brain barrier—designed to keep your neurological function safe from harm. Once inside, mercury can damage both the neurons which transmit information throughout your brain and the myelin sheaths that surround them.

How might mercury have been causing the facial palsy that Bell and others began to see? If you trace the tiny end points of the cranial nerves all the way back into your brain stem, you will find that they originate from neuronal tissue referred to as *cranial nerve nuclei—* nuclei is plural for *nucleus*. Each cranial nerve, (remember there are often pairs of them—one for each side) has its own nucleus—a control center that issues commands for movement from the brain in the case of motor nerves, or conveys sensation to the brain in the case of sensory nerves.

If you look for images of the nuclei, you won't find many photos but instead illustrations—hand-drawn depictions of oblong blobs that look like distinctly colored glands or tiny organs. They are actually *indistinct* portions of neuronal matter within the brain stem and can be difficult to distinguish from each other. This is why you won't often find photographs of cranial nerve nuclei—they're not very photogenic. They are camouflaged and cannot easily be snipped out with a scalpel for dissection like a lymph node or a spleen. It is only through exhaustive research that the location and sizes of these different cranial nerve control centers have come to be known.

When tissue within your body gets damaged, we call these lesions. Your body is usually able to heal itself perfectly, but the neuronal pathways in your brain can be much more tricky. When you develop a lesion in your brain, the pathways that are damaged—either through the neurons or myelin sheaths—attempt to reconnect to each other. Sometimes, they miss.

If you've ever watched time lapse photography of a vine growing, you will have seen little tendrils shooting off the vine and curling around whatever they touch. Sometimes, the tendrils shoot into thin air and cannot connect with anything. When parts of your brain become damaged, they attempt to reconnect with each other, just like tendrils from the vine. Sometimes they are able to reconnect properly and their original function can be restored. Other times, they do not and may become permanently useless.

When neurotoxins like mercury cause neuronal damage, the brain will lose function because the pathway is interrupted. It will attempt to heal itself, and if the original damage was minimal, enough connections may reform so that the basic functionality is regained. If the damage is severe, the likelihood for complete repair is very low—there will be too many "misses" as the neuronal pathways attempt to reconnect.

When a motor neuron pathway is damaged, your ability to enervate the muscles on the end of that nerve is weakened. There may be enough strands to create some movement, but with an imperfect connection, it will be evident through muscle weakness. An eye may drift outward. A smile may become lopsided. With concentration, some of these deficiencies can be corrected, but the natural state will exhibit asymmetry.

There are many other functions within the brain that can be damaged by mercury, as was evidenced by the gruesome "thick deposits of coagulable lymph" and other strange effects visible in autopsied brains of the day. Although tiny amounts of mercury were certainly capable of causing lesions in the cranial nerve nuclei that controlled facial and eye muscles, their proximity to other cranial nerve nuclei meant that more wide-ranging injury was certain to occur.

TORTICOLLIS

I had been researching crooked faces for over a year when a random connection appeared again. Although I didn't realize it at the time, a single image would transform a simple search for the cause of crooked faces into a much larger journey.

I was scrolling through a collection of pictures when I saw a baby wearing a helmet. The image initially struck me because the baby had an obvious crooked smile—up on the right, down on the left. The helmet wasn't a bicycle helmet, but a corrective one with cartoons on it. I'd seen them before, but weren't quite sure what they were for.

I looked up why babies sometimes wear helmets: *Plagiocephaly*—an asymmetrical head shape triggered by a variety of things, cause often unknown. The human skull is formed from several loosely connected cranial bones that fuse over time. Until then, the infant head is a malleable thing and can be easily deformed. Plagiocephaly rates have increased lately, possibly due in part to the "Back to Sleep" programs aimed at cutting down on SIDS rates.[16] Back-sleeping associated plagiocephaly tends to create a flattened shape on the back of the head.

Other types of plagiocephaly can create asymmetrical shapes that tend to be more visible from the top of the skull than the side. And for some reason, these other types of deformities are often associated with a phenomenon called *torticollis*.

It is suggested that torticollis appears in babies when one of their neck muscles is shorter than the other. Some babies appear to be born with it, although their lack of muscle tone at such a young age makes a diagnosis difficult. Torticollis often appears just months after birth and is clearly noticeable because a baby will tilt their head significantly to one side. This warped pose places additional weight on one side of their yet-to-fuse skull bones and creates an abnormal growth pattern that can be set right with a corrective helmet.

As I began looking through images of babies with torticollis-associated plagiocephaly, crooked faces began popping up. It was remarkable how frequently they appeared. As always, I suspected my bias was coloring the observation so I looked through the scientific literature to see if anyone else had noticed. To my surprise, asymmetrical faces were commonly mentioned alongside torticollis.[17] Studies had even been conducted to observe whether torticollis treatments corrected facial asymmetry.[18] It wasn't just me—even scientists had also noticed that crooked faces were a common occurrence among babies with torticollis.

A quick survey revealed a fascinating phenomenon I had already noticed in the way people seemed to smile. The babies heads seemed to favor tilting towards the right side. There were some towards to the left, but I realized many of these images featured the hand of a parent, therapeutically pulling the child's head in that direction in an attempt to strengthen the weaker side of their neck. In other words, many of these left-tilting images were showing ways to *correct* torticollis. If there was a weakness on the left side of the baby's neck, the weight of their head would tend to pull it to their right. Just like with smiles, these babies tended to show left side paralysis.

I came across another study that confused me at the time but proved remarkably insightful later: Children with plagiocephaly as infants were associated with developmental delays. According to the study, "25 of the 63 children (39.7%) with persistent deformational plagiocephaly had received special help in primary school including: special education assistance, physical therapy, occupational therapy, speech therapy generally through an Individual Education Plan. Only 7 of 91 siblings (7.7%), serving as controls, required similar services."[19] Could a slightly misshapen brain actually cause learning disorders? I wasn't sure what to make of the study, but logged it anyway and hoped that perhaps it would make sense later.

Some of the research I had read suggested that facial asymmetry in babies with torticollis might just be an effect of gravity. Because the head was often tilted, maybe the additional weight on one side of the face was causing asymmetry. So I began to look for studies on torticollis and strabismus. I thought surely a tilted head couldn't cause people's eyes to become misaligned. What some of the research suggested was very surprising.

Strabismus was associated with torticollis, but it was implied that torticollis was *because* of the strabismus, not just associated with it.[20] Most strabismus typically involves a lateral deviation of one eye—it is out of alignment to the left or right. Occasionally, you will see vertical misalignment problems. The resulting double vision can be corrected to an extent by tilting the head. Although this type of strabismus is rare, the concept was an interesting side note to the exploration.

According to my theory, problems with the 7th cranial nerve could cause the crooked smile, and problems with the 3rd, 4th or 6th cranial nerves could cause misaligned eyes. But a tilted neck? Could torticollis actually be caused by the same thing that was causing crooked faces?

The possibility of a common link between more than just the smile and eyes was exhilarating, but I suspected it probably would not be true.

I wasn't familiar enough with anatomy to understand how the head moved, so I looked through some illustrations and saw there are mainly two pairs of muscles controlling the head: the *trapezius* muscles on the back of the neck, and the *sternocleidomastoid* muscles on the front. There are a few minor muscles underneath, but these are the four main ones that allow you to swivel your head around.

Torticollis didn't fit the cranial nerve theory—it wasn't something in the brain or face. It was the actual body, something to do with the shoulder or neck muscles. I looked for an illustration of which nerves controlled those muscles, thinking they would have to originate near the top of the spinal column. I was shocked when I realized these four muscles were controlled by the accessory nerve, also called the 11th cranial nerve.

A problem with the 11th cranial nerve on one side could create weakness in those two muscles—the ones that held the head upright. If the muscles on one side of the neck weren't working properly, the head would tilt the other way—just like with the eyes. When both muscles on the sides of the eye worked in tandem, they kept it centered. When one side was weak, the eye would deviate away from it.

The game of connect-the-dots that had been floating in my mind grew exponentially bigger. The overlap was undeniable—people with crooked smiles sometimes had strabismus. And people with torticollis often had crooked smiles *and* strabismus. If the 3rd, 4th, 7th and 11th cranial nerves could develop palsy from the same thing, there was no reason why all the cranial nerves couldn't be affected. Whatever might be causing these cranial nerve palsies had just turned into a real monster.

BELL'S FOURTH CASE

It had become clear to me that it wasn't just crooked smiles and misaligned eyes—the same thing causing cranial nerve palsies of the face and eyes might also affect any of the other cranial nerves. If the tilted heads of torticollis and their plagiocephaly helmets were indeed just more examples of cranial nerve asymmetry, then shouldn't there be examples of other cranial nerve problems? And if so, shouldn't we be able to find examples in medical literature from around this same time period?

It took one final case from Charles Bell's presentation to answer both of these questions.

No. XVIII
Case of Periodical Blindness, from a Cause not hitherto observed.

"The subject of this case is a young lady, twenty-four years of age, of delicate frame, with great intelligence and expression;

accomplished, and, as ladies are, studious. She was in the habit of drawing a great deal, and had painted a miniature a short time before the symptoms I have to describe commenced. In giving the case, I am assisted by the letter of her physician, which she presented to me, and which shows that he has studied the symptoms, having that interest in the case which is so naturally excited in a benevolent mind.

In August, 1826, she began to have headaches, which, however, had not a common character: the pain extended down the side of her face to the angle of the jaw, and then backwards into the ear, with a sensation of tightness in the skin of the forehead; and this pain she had first on one and then on the other side of her face. These pains appeared to her physician to be 'connected with considerable disorder of her stomach and alimentary canal, increased, if not produced, by too sedentary a habit, and application to drawing. After a dose of calomel and opium, she took, in succession, the sulphate of quinine, the extract of henbane, and the liquor arsenicalis. She had also the blue pill, until her mouth became a little sore.'

The pain had ceased, and a 'heavy stupidness,' to use her own expression, prevailed for a few days; when one day, in reading, she found that she could not see the letters,—they were thrown together and confounded. This obscurity of vision was attended with a fluttering in the eyes, which seemed to her alternately to open and shut with great rapidity; by turning away from her book and attending to other things, she could read for some time, when she again looked upon the page. The application of leeches relieved these symptoms for a day or two; but the relief was temporary, and she gradually lost the power of directing her eyes. From the beginning of this affection of the eyes, the pain ceased in the head. This 'actual blindness came on periodically. It began about ten o'clock in the morning and ceased about four; and, during the blindness, there was constantly presented a most quick motion of the eye-lids and eye-balls; and, during the whole of these attacks, she lost all control over the muscles of the eye-lids and eye balls. She could partly see, or at least distinguish light from darkness.' Her vision was occasionally restored: at one time her medical man having made his visit he was called back as he was stepping into his carriage, she having at that moment entirely recovered her sight. Her blindness has of late been permanent.

…This young lady has a pleasant, intelligent manner : but I observed to her, that she conversed with her ears! on which she said, 'Oh dear, am I already so bad as that?' understanding perfectly what I meant, –that the direction of her countenance to those who addressed her was like that of a blind person.

…The secretion of tears flows plentifully. There is not the slightest degree of inflammation in the eyes … She, however, adds, 'I wonder, considering the many questions you put to me yesterday, that I forgot a circumstance which is, perhaps, important; that I have pain extending round the head as if it were bound by a hoop. This is not continual, but is excited by the motion of a carriage or by noise. I have also,' said she, 'a whizzing noise in my ears, especially when I awake in the morning.'"[21]

Mercury wasn't the only problem affecting people during this time. Due to the advance of the Industrial Revolution, other metallic compounds began finding their way into our bodies.

A new compound called copper acetate triarsenate was invented in 1814. Although it would later become a popular insecticide and pesticide due to its toxicity, the substance was originally used as a color pigment. The brilliant new dye—known as "Paris Green"—was an instant hit amongst painters, wallpaper manufacturers, furniture makers, toy companies and even bakers and confectionary shops, who would use it to color their cakes and candies. The arsenic trioxide component of Paris Green may have been just as toxic as the arsenical solutions being administered by physicians of the day, possibly more so due to it being inadvertently inhaled rather than ingested. Undoubtedly, patients who became ill from the fumes of this toxic color dye would receive "treatment" in the form of more arsenic or mercury. It was not a good time to be sick.

In Bell's account, the young woman clearly attributed painting to the onset of her sickness: pain throughout her head and an unspecified gut issue—something we can presume was constipation. Paris Green, though not specified, would be an obvious suspect in the cause of her mysterious headaches and abdominal pain following her artistic endeavors. Early on, no one suspected the emerald green paint might be dangerous. Even seventy years later in the 1890s, when a chemist determined the mysterious cause of death for a group of a thousand Italian children to be the fumes from Paris Green infused wallpaper, few believed him.[22]

This twenty-four year old woman paid an innocent visit to the local physician who prescribed her opium, calomel (a mercury compound), liquor arsenicalis—also known as Fowler's solution (a liquid containing a form of arsenic)—and for good measure was given "blue pills", another mercuric medicine. Unsurprisingly, her issues became worse. She developed what she called a "heavy stupidness"—what we can imagine would now be described as brain fog. The account then mentions that she found that she couldn't read, because "she could not see the letters,– they were thrown together and confounded," a condition that sounds like *diplopia*—double vision, possibly caused by a sudden onset of strabismus.

New symptoms developed, such as partial blindness alongside rapid uncontrollable blinking—something which we might call facial *tics*. Leeches were tried without success. In addition to problems with her eyelids, her eyes "constantly presented a most quick motion," an early reference to something we might call *nystagmus*.[i]

The entire listing of her many symptoms contained another curious tidbit: She would direct her ears towards the speaker rather than her eyes, as if she had trouble hearing what they said. But at the same time she had headaches that were exacerbated by the motion of riding in a carriage or by noise. She mentioned she would wake up to a whizzing noise in her ears.

This woman's condition, possibly triggered initially by the inhalation of arsenic via Paris Green fumes, then worsened by the administration of mercury and yet more arsenic (in the form of Fowler's solution), lacks the tell-tale description of the crooked face. But her symptoms suggested that besides the typical afflictions of acute metal toxicity, other cranial nerves had been affected, specifically the 8th cranial nerve—the *vestibulocochlear* nerve.

Problems with the 8th cranial nerve can create issues with hearing and motion. The woman began to experience discomfort from the movement of riding in a horse-drawn carriage—perhaps an early form of motion sensitivity. The rapid eye movement her doctor described—nystagmus—can also be attributed to problems with her vestibular system. Tilting her ears towards a voice in order to better understand them while at the same time complaining of loud noises resembles the symptoms of a common definition of *hyperacusis*: an increased sensitivity to certain frequencies and volumes of sound coupled with a difficulty in separating foreground noises from background noises. Certain noises become agonizingly loud, while others become difficult to discern. After some moderate improvement, she attempted to venture out, into a crowded event: "She enjoyed one night at the play, but returned from it with a severe headache, fell into bad health and

---

i. A vision condition where the eye makes rapid, involuntary movements, most often side to side. Interestingly, the rapid eye movements of her eyelids and eyes seemed to abate, at least temporarily, after opiate treatments.

bad spirits…"[23]

One cannot read these descriptions of her symptoms and behavior and not be reminded of modern day SPD, or *sensory processing disorder*, an affliction often occurring alongside autism. SPD spans a wide range of symptoms, from texture sensitivities to an intense dislike of change and is an absolutely horrible affliction, if only because most can't understand why (or sometimes believe) the afflicted is actually suffering. If this woman were alive today, her hearing sensitivities, coupled with motion sensitivity and nystagmus would probably have gotten her an SPD diagnosis and a visit to the occupational therapist.

The young lady's condition never seemed to improve and a somber note ended the description of her case: "…she has recovered her spirits, and, by opening the eyelids of one eye, the other eye is disclosed also; and in a moderate degree she can enjoy her reading and drawing."[24] We can only hope she was indeed drawing, and not painting.

Although impossible to verify, it would appear that in the early 1800s metal toxicity from either mercury or arsenic was entirely capable of creating problems in the 3rd, 4th, 6th, 7th and now 8th cranial nerves. Was there more cranial nerve dysfunction hidden amongst Bell's 89 cases? Regardless, the net I had originally cast using crooked smiles and misaligned eyes as its criteria was spreading out much further than I had ever thought possible.

PULL TO SIT

I was reading through some research on gait[i] asymmetry in autism when I remembered a news story with Diane Sawyer. It had been years ago when the nightly network news outlets still broke big stories before the internet. They all seemed to cover this one: a new test allowed early detection of autism—something that everyone had been searching for in vain. With nothing but dead-ends coming from genetic testing, the general public is always happy to hear something positive about the autism epidemic overtaking our children (1 in 36 at last count[25]).

The test was based on a study that looked at 40 babies with brothers diagnosed with ASD.[26] Ninety percent of those that failed the test would go on to be diagnosed with autism spectrum disorder. Another group looked at 22 babies and found that 75% of the children with ASD failed the test. It was a remarkably accurate test to be conducted at such a young age (6, 14 or 24 months) and able to predict an autism diagnosis over a year or two later. For many parents, when no other signs of

---

i. The pattern in which one walks or runs.

issues were present in their children, this presented a promising way to screen your children for potential signs of autism long before it was otherwise detectable.

What was this incredible test? It was called the Pull-To-Sit test and was something any parent could do in the comfort of their home without any training from a medical professional. To conduct the test, the baby was laid on their back, feet towards the parent. The parent would grasp both babies hands and gently pull them into a sitting position. If the baby's body came up evenly, with their head aligned with their torso, it indicated that everything was likely okay. If their head did not come up with their body—what researchers referred to as *head lag*—this indicated a problem.

In that initial test within the study, 90% of babies whose head lagged behind their body as they were being pulled into a sitting position would go on to be diagnosed with autism, months or even years later. Weak head and neck control were mentioned in story after story as potential indicators of neurological development issues beyond autism, but no one seemed to have any idea why.

If you put your hand under your jaw and push down hard with your chin, you will feel two muscles on the sides of your neck flex. These are the sternocleidomastoid muscles, and if you remember what was said about torticollis, they are controlled by the 11th cranial nerve, the *accessory* nerve. Here was a new study that went beyond anything I could have asked for and found a very distinct marker for autism— head lag when being pulled into a sitting position. About the only thing that could reliably trigger muscle weakness in the sternocleidomastoid muscles was a problem with the 11th cranial nerve.

Later, during my research to try and understand *postural orthostatic tachycardia syndrome* (POTS), I would come to realize that babies who failed the test might also have problems with their 8th vestibulocochlear nerve as well. This cranial nerve determines our sense of balance and orientation and if the inner ear isn't working properly, it can prevent multiple reflexes from occurring during posture changes—reflexes that determine head positioning in relation to the body.

I pounded my fists on my desk in frustration. They were missing two obvious causes for children failing this Pull-To-Sit test. And if they were missing this, there was no doubt in my mind they were also missing crooked faces along with all the other cranial nerves. If a palsy on the 8th or 11th cranial nerve could be a potential warning sign for autism, then so could the others—the misaligned eyes. The crooked mouths. And everything else.

MOTOR & SENSORY NERVES

Another interesting phenomenon began to occur to me. Remember there are two types of nerves—motor and sensory. The motor nerves are what conduct commands from your brain to your muscles for movement, and the sensory nerves are what receive inputs from various places in your body. They allow you to feel textures, smell, see, hear, taste. Even beyond the basic senses, they allow feedback between various organs in your body, notably between your gut and your brain —one of the most fascinating and least understood communication networks in your body.

When motor nerves develop a problem, the muscles they control weaken. They receive fewer impulses for motion, which causes them to move less, an effect that is exacerbated over time. If you develop a lesion on one of your 7th cranial nerve branches, the muscles it controls will be less powerful—they will not be able to contract fully and you will see it show up as asymmetry on the face. If your 12th cranial nerve develops a lesion, some of the muscles that control your tongue will be weaker and forming the complex shapes that allow human speech will become suddenly difficult.

For reasons unknown, when your sensory nerves develop problems, the opposite effect often happens. The organs which they are connected to exhibit *hypersensitivity*. Some cranial *motor* nerve palsies can be an annoyance, but cranial *sensory* nerve palsies can be hell on earth. Whisper quiet sounds that you can't ignore. Ordinary textures that feel worse than nails on a chalkboard. The slightest motions overwhelm. Imagine these sensitivities played out within the vagus nerve and its connection to the endocrine system and you can imagine why behavioral and sleep issues might be considered a hallmark of cranial nerve palsies.

Throughout all of my research, I believed that I had steered clear of any cranial nerve palsies, besides possibly a weak-sided smile I occasionally exhibit. But as I learned more about the sensory issues with cranial nerve lesions, I began to think I was perhaps mistaken.

In the early 2000s, I was doing a lot of video and animation work for the Discovery Health Channel, working on shows like "The Duggars" and "John and Kate Plus 8." We would often go out to eat lunch with the producers of the show and inevitably they noticed something about me, like most people had my entire life.

"You eat like a 4-year-old," they would tell me.

"Are you seriously going to eat that like that?" another person would ask.

"Yes and yes," I would tell them, having developed very thick skin over years of being teased—from both my quirky name and my quirky eating habits.

I *did* eat like a 4-year-old and I *was* going to eat like that. It had been going on since I could remember. I wanted everything *plain*. Cheese was an advanced topping for me, something I would only be able to add to my repertoire later on in childhood. I didn't want pepper on my potato. I didn't want salt on my grits and I certainly didn't want butter on my pancakes. I wanted anything with carbohydrates and nothing in between it and my mouth. Doritos felt like they were burning holes in my tongue. Dr. Pepper made me want to vomit.

And it wasn't just taste. It was textures. Corn on the cob I could deal with. Corn *off* the cob, in a bowl—I would starve before I'd eat it. Cooked vegetables were out of the question. Boiled okra, no. Green beans, no. Anything with multiple conflicting textures like casserole was torture.

If any of you reading this have witnessed this behavior in your children, you know how maddening it is to try and go anywhere with your child and keep them alive with the offense that is food. My poor mother didn't understand why I was being so difficult, and my 7-year-old self certainly had no idea, considering my 46-year-old self is just now figuring it out.

The Discovery Health Channel producers came up with an idea—they thought a documentary about my eating habits would be entertaining, and wanted to film me over the course of a year as they sent me around to various places to try and cure my problem.

There were the usual suspects—a hardcore personal trainer who made sure to point out the orange vomit buckets before our first workout (I refused the orange bucket and used the bathroom instead). There was a fancy nutritionist from Duke Hospital who spent an hour with me and grew increasingly disheartened as she went through a giant Excel spreadsheet of foods, crossing them off the list one by one.

"You're going to have to try some new things if you want to eat healthier," she said.

"New things?" That was my cue to leave. I hated new things. I wanted the same thing. Every day. No surprises.

I was taken to the first of several sessions with the head of the Duke University Eating Disorder Clinic. She specialized in children with "food aversion", something I'd never heard of but felt described me correctly—both the aversion and the child descriptor. The girls in the waiting room must have had a field day trying to diagnose my ailment.[i]

Within minutes, the doctor had diagnosed me with OCD, which was probably half-right. Therapy, medicine and meditation were in order and would help. I tried to explain that I was a "Super taster" and had done a test where I counted the number of taste buds on my tongue and the density was higher than a normal person—something that might explain why Doritos burned my mouth. But she wouldn't have it—it was therapy, anxiety control through meditation, and possibly medication in the form of Celexa.

I wasn't sure the medicine was even working at all until I was on a business trip in Vancouver and my host asked me if he could take me out for sushi.

"Sure," I said, amazed at the lack of spine-tingling anxiety I was expecting when having to confront the possibility of eating adult foods.

We went to a fancy restaurant where I confessed to him I'd never tried sushi before. He went on to explain the different types of sushi, from mild to wild.

"Sashimi," he said. "That's hardcore if you've never tried it. Totally raw."

"Sashimi!" I said with profound shock. "Let's DO IT!"

I couldn't believe my newfound powers. Eventually, the side effects of the anti-anxiety medicine would end up being too much for me to deal with, but before I weaned myself off, it revealed one more surprise. I was in the bedroom closet getting ready for work and reached for a pair of pants. Not shorts, but pants.

You may have seen a meme floating around the internet that depicts a guy in shorts in the snow with the caption, "There's always that one guy." I was that guy—to the most infinite extreme you can imagine. I didn't wear pants ever in high school, except possibly my

---

i. I do not cut a slight figure.

graduation ceremony. I would snow ski in shorts if I could bear it. My entire professional career arc had been guided not by salary, benefits or working conditions, but whether I had to wear pants or not. Like my eating habits, it was a constant embarrassment I could not explain to anyone.

I had tried to explain it to my mother, who insisted I wear pants to school on colder days. They constricted me and they were uncomfortable. It felt like they grated on my legs and I couldn't think about anything other than when I would be able to get them off. I originally attributed it to having an abnormal body shape but was assured by the salesmen at J.C. Penney that Levis 501 jeans fit me correctly.

It wasn't until recently, as I studied the hypersensitivities of sensory processing disorder and autistic children, that I would recognize some of these same traits in myself. If you don't know it already, clothing can be a very difficult issue for some of these children. Tags feel like horseflies. Corduroy, like barbed wire. Denim, like sandpaper. Thankfully, there are now clothing companies dedicated to making compression vests and other SPD friendly clothing.

Looking back on my lifetime of food and pants aversion—the texture issues and extreme sensitivity to the slightest of tastes and touches—I can't help but wonder if I also developed a 7th or possibly 9th cranial nerve palsy, sometime as a child. [ii]

---

ii. The show would finish and air in 2004-2005 on Discovery Health Channel under the name "Ultimate Body Challenge: Forrest's Story." It would occasionally re-air on FitTV. The food aversions, though less pronounced than they were ten years ago still exist. Still never tried coffee, and I'm not wearing pants.

AUTISM & ASYMMETRY

Another remarkable overlap became apparent. Many of the children I had seen with crooked faces had ASD (*autism spectrum disorder*). It wasn't always, but it was there—a common pattern I couldn't ignore. A slight sideways smile that was neither smirk nor grin. Eye gazes that felt subtly soft instead of razor sharp. In fact, I felt I could sometimes detect if a child had ASD simply by observing their face. While this ability may sound like some physiognomic parlor trick, I have spoken to parents of autistic children who claim Spiderman-like abilities at divining other children on the spectrum while they are out and about.

"I can always tell," one mother told me. "It's a sixth sense. I don't need to see hand-flapping or finger-clicking. It's just immediate. I can spot it a mile away. I don't think I've ever been wrong."

Another mom confided, "I wonder if they see it in my son like I do theirs. I want to go up to them and talk to them—you know, give them a hug, because we're in this together, but it's like if someone's pregnant. You think they're pregnant, and want to say something nice, but you don't want to be wrong."

Identifying someone's mental state based purely on their appearance was something Charles Bell and many other scientists had discussed, so I began to look for scientific support for this ability. Although abnormalities within the facial structure had been used to predict neurological issues,[27] I never suspected facial asymmetry might indicate autism. Children with ASD seem to develop completely normally—with very few signs of anything wrong. While there are some neurological issues that may be visible to the naked eye, autism didn't seem like one of them.

Even if one were to peer into the genetic code that created a child with ASD, they would find little unique—the most commonly occurring single gene disorder in autism, Fragile X, appears in only 5% of cases, and only 30% of children with Fragile X develop it.[28] Other research indicates that many genetic mutations associated with ASD were not present in the children's parents, appearing *de novo* in the affected child. This would implicate an environmental cause for the mutation, something which might exponentially complicate the autism riddle.[29][i]

Surprisingly, there had been a very thorough look into facial symmetry in ASD. The study was called "Face–brain asymmetry in autism spectrum disorders"[30] and it used 3-dimensional computer modeling technology to map the facial morphology of 72 boys with ASD, 128 of their first-degree relatives, and 254 unrelated controls. This study was particularly fascinating to me because up until that point, all my observations had been decidedly unscientific. Completely biased and useless to anyone but myself.

The researchers employed sophisticated computer vision to mathematically determine asymmetry without the bias of knowing

---

i. Unfortunately, the search for genetic clues to autism, despite over 20 years of searching and hundreds of millions of dollars in research has so far been of little use in its prevention or possible recovery.

which faces belonged to those who had been diagnosed with ASD. The results were remarkable. Those with ASD showed marked asymmetry compared to the control group (those with no ASD diagnosis). Using the 3d mapping data alongside pattern matching software, they were able to predict if someone had autism, based on specific asymmetry in their face—with 82% accuracy.

You can imagine the revelation this study was to me. It was a very thorough, data-driven look at facial asymmetry in autism with no possibility for interference from interpretive bias that I could find, and it was fairly conclusive: Boys with ASD showed significant facial asymmetry—enough that a computer could separate them out from non-ASD faces 82% of the time.

As I read through the study a second and third time, something occurred to me: the study didn't look at eye alignment—it was just the face. This was a significant data point that was left out of the study. If they would have been able to take into account asymmetry by also using eye alignment, it would be safe to assume the accuracy would have gone up. How far up? 85%? 90%? Even without taking into account the eyes, the results seemed promising.

But then something disheartening occurred to me: Not only was this study not looking at eye alignment, it wasn't actually looking at muscles at all. It was looking at bone structure. They weren't testing the range of motion of people's smiles—nothing that might indicate cranial nerve palsy. The data was generated from 3d scans of people's faces, after which 18 "landmark" points, such as the inside corners of their eyes, were carefully tagged. It represented the bone structure of their face, and seemed to have nothing to do with proper cranial nerve function.

I was about to catalog the paper in the "Re-examine Later" folder, but another finding from the study caught my eye: Right side asymmetrical dominance.

>"We conclude that previously identified right dominant asymmetry of the frontal poles of boys with ASD could explain their facial asymmetry through the direct effect of brain growth … Shape difference is then visibly detectable in the supraorbital, nasal, zygomatic and perioral regions, especially on the right side … This confirmed the right supraorbital and zygomatic dominance … provided additional evidence of right dominant asymmetry for the ASD boys…"[31]

Here it was. I had noticed that more of the crooked smiles seemed to be up on the right, down on the left. I had noticed that more of the babies with torticollis tilted their head to the right instead of the left. But these were just my hack observations, with not even an Excel spreadsheet to show for it. Here was scientific evidence—computer generated data points, no less—that indicated the 72 subjects with ASD in this study showed a marked asymmetrical dominance on a particular side—the right side.

For a moment, I was jubilant. My observations of facial asymmetry favoring a particular side weren't just in my mind—they actually existed. Something was causing this asymmetry to favor one side over the other. I had no idea what, but it was something—a tiny confirmation of something potentially huge. But then I remembered the study was looking at bone structure. Nothing to do with cranial nerves. And the research indicated the asymmetry was on the *right* side. Everything I had noticed before indicated that the palsy was on the left side, not the right. My mind swam with confusion for days as I tried to reckon the apparent conflict. Months later, the answer to this riddle would come from an unlikely source—a book on polio.

EVEN THE BONES?

There was one more finding from the "Face–brain asymmetry in autism spectrum disorders" research that struck me. The scientists didn't just study the faces of 72 boys with ASD, they also studied their parents. And by using the same 3d mapping and pattern matching algorithms, they were able to predict if a mother had a child with ASD with 76% accuracy. Not perfect, but still, a significant number within a very odd discovery: Particular facial asymmetry in the mother alone could be used to predict ASD in her children with a fair degree of certainty. It wasn't perfect, but yet—there was something there. Perhaps the women I spoke with weren't just basing their autism detection on what the children looked like. They may have unknowingly been analyzing the children's mothers as well.

I was still confused by the apparent right-side dominant facial asymmetry seen in the study. Everything I had observed indicated that left side palsy was more common. Yet they seemed to have noticed the opposite? It didn't make sense to me.

The inconsistency drove me absolutely crazy for the next few months until a clue popped up in some research I was doing on paralytic diseases of the late 1800s and 1900s.[i] If you've ever seen pictures of people suffering the effects of "Infantile Paralysis," as polio was originally called, you will have no doubt noticed the withered legs and horribly contorted bodies. How does a disease that paralyses cause such terrible deformities?

Many of the motions your body can perform are the result of two offsetting muscle groups—one to extend and the other to retract. The *peroneus* muscles on the front of your shin are smaller and are used to lift the front of your foot up (imagine "lifting off the gas" in a car) while the much larger *gastrocnemius* muscle on the back of your calf is used to lift the back of your foot up (and the weight of your entire body along with it). If you were to develop paralysis in the front of your shin, you would not be able to lift the front of your foot and the offsetting muscle would dominate. If the paralysis did not go away, the muscle would atrophy and your foot would develop a permanent deformity—in this case, the *equinus* position (where the foot points downward) that is common amongst paralysis victims. Like the deviations caused by strabismus, if there is an imbalance in two opposing muscle groups, paralysis may cause a permanent deviation.

However, a second problem occurs with paralysis, this one more relevant to our facial asymmetry discussion. Bones don't just randomly get bigger—they grow in part according to the demand placed upon them by muscles attached to them. If a bone on the left side of your body were to have no muscle attached to it, demanding nothing of it, it would not grow in the same way as the identical bone on the right side of your body—with an active muscle attached to it.

Because of this, you may see disturbing pictures of young paralytic children with horrible spine curvatures. The muscles that support their torso may have been paralyzed on one side and as a result their spine is

---

i. I'm writing a book on the fascinating story of polio called "The Moth in the Iron Lung."

curved towards the good side as it makes more demands than the other. Even the most stout of bones can grow strangely if, over time, a little uneven pressure is added.

The same phenomenon happens with our head and even our face. The skull is divided into two parts—the *neurocranium* which surrounds your brain, and the *viscerocranium* which makes up your face and jaw. Like the neurocranium, your viscerocranium is made up of several different bones that are loosely attached by fibrous joints called *sutures*. The resulting plasticity is what makes plagiocephaly (a deformed head shape) possible. Over time, these sutures fuse to create a more rigid skull. Interestingly, some of the *neuro* sutures begin to fuse within two years of birth. Other sutures, such as some of those on your face, don't fully fuse until 20, even 30 years of age. In addition to the fickle expansion of bone, these unformed sutures make the forming of your skull subject to the whims of the muscles that pull on them.

Having observed the contorted shapes that paralytic children grow into, and understanding how unbalanced muscle tension can twist the growth of a bone into unimaginable forms, it wasn't hard to see how the face—and the actual bone structure underneath—might become distorted over time with facial palsy.

If the skull structure of ASD children was going to display differences from the control group, it would make sense that these distortions might appear on the half where there was increased tension —the only half where the muscles were working at full strength. And in my observation, this was often the right side. This is where we should *expect* to see structural changes to the bone.

With my enthusiasm for the study renewed, I pulled the "Face-brain asymmetry" paper out and took a closer look at the 3-d images detailing specific locations of asymmetry. The regions they illustrated having right-side dominance were the *supraorbital* (just above the eye), the *perioral* (around the mouth) and the *zygomatic* (below the outer side of the eye).

A quick look at the muscles of the face revealed the answer. The zygomaticus muscles originate underneath the supraorbital region and *insert* (or end) at the *orbicularis oris*, the muscles around the mouth. These muscles have a very specific purpose—they're what allow you to smile. In a face where the muscles on the right side are functioning at full strength and the left are not, we might expect to see more skeletal asymmetry on the right side. This study confirmed exactly what I had noticed – more often, people seemed to experience paralysis on the left side of their face and retain function on their right.

Although I was ecstatic at having a scientific study confirm my observations, I was faced with uncovering the obvious question—Why? Why was the paralysis often on the left side instead of the right? The answer to that question would not come until many months later as I began to understand the way in which metal moves throughout our body.

If you have some time to read through the paper, you should. The 3-d renderings are colored green on the face where there was no difference between the ASD facial structure and the controls. They're colored blue where the geometry of the skull deviated out away from where it was in the control group, and red where it deviated inward. With these simple illustrations, you can easily imagine the effects that the pushing and pulling of various facial muscles might have on the skull over time.

The paper may actually present a fascinating look into subtle morphological distinctions of not only autism, but cranial nerve damage as well. If pattern-matching algorithms can guess ASD faces correctly with 82% accuracy, then mothers, with many more data points available to them (body posture, gait, eye alignment, etc.) combined with human's incredible facial recognition abilities—perhaps they really do have superhuman abilities to detect autism.

IT'S ALL OF THEM

Although it had been described over 200 years earlier by Charles Bell, during the height of "Heroic" medicine, something special happened recently to cause the numbers of people with crooked faces to flourish. I was fairly certain the asymmetry had a tendency to occur on the left side. I had a very thorough study that had confirmed it. I had no idea why it might be happening, but it was a pattern I had recognized informally and was able to confirm with scientific data.

With proof crooked faces were more common in children with ASD, I began to take stock of other diseases that might show a prevalence of asymmetry. It was apparent that facial palsy was associated with others: Guillan-Barré syndrome, Rett syndrome, Moebius syndrome, Parry Romberg, Myasthenia gravis, Ptosis, Otitis media facial palsy, and Lyme-induced facial palsy. As I looked closer, it seemed as though an asymmetrical face was part and parcel of many other diseases. A good deal of the people I noticed with Alzheimer's, ALS, Multiple sclerosis, Parkinson's, even Gardasil-related paralysis—they had crooked grins or misaligned eyes. And in a disturbing discovery, I looked through pictures of people who had died from the flu vaccine, and even children who had died of SIDS—many of them also had crooked faces.

And I couldn't help but remember Joshua, who had nearly lost his life to seizures and was now diagnosed with autism. My wife, just after she developed Crohn's, and Robert with hyperacusis—they all showed signs of facial palsy. It was a remarkable coincidence I couldn't ignore.

I was beginning to believe there might be a common thread I was missing. If all of these different diseases featured various forms of facial palsy, then perhaps they all had a common origin. An even more unlikely idea began to form in my head: Maybe, all these illnesses—the ones where crooked faces popped up so frequently—maybe they weren't separate disorders at all, but were in fact symptoms of the same illness? A single disease—with many different symptoms—that began to surface over two hundred years ago during the Heroic era of medicinal metals, but had now taken on a slightly different form.

Perhaps mercury's delirium had become today's autism and Alzheimer's. Perhaps yesterday's gastritis had become today's Crohn's and ulcerative colitis. Was it possible that both the older and modern diseases—even the autoimmune and neurological disorders that were not prevalent until the last fifty or sixty years—were all caused by the same thing? Variations on a terrible theme?

IN SEARCH OF AUTOIMMUNITY

It seemed that metals, particularly those administered for medicinal purposes, were creating the crooked faces of yesteryear—just like they do today. I suspected that many of the autoimmune disorders now so prevalent might also be triggered by metal toxicity. If that was the case, we should be able to find autoimmune disorders two hundred years ago. They wouldn't look exactly the same because they were likely caused by different metals. They certainly wouldn't be called "autoimmune" because our knowledge of the immune system, even our ability to see anything smaller than bacteria, was so primitive the concept couldn't have existed. But I thought they would be there—in some form. Hidden from plain view, just like our faces.

I searched for months through the old medical literature for signs of various autoimmune diseases: inflammatory bowel diseases, fibromyalgia, chronic fatigue. There were mentions of symptoms that resembled components of these various disorders, but no common link —no sense of an over-arching pattern of illness that might be yesteryear's autoimmune disease.

I was halfway through writing this book and had given up hope of finding it when a very curious phrase appeared in an old work on *neurasthenia* I was reading. Neurasthenia appeared in the medical literature in the early 1800s as a term to describe a neurological condition that many people had recently begun to suffer from. Its symptoms appeared to be linked to the central nervous system—fatigue, exhaustion, mood disorders, headaches—and was thought to have been the result of the stresses of "modern" living. The United States was apparently so modernized the condition was even jokingly called "Americanitis."[32]

Neurasthenia's wide variety of neurological symptoms defied explanation and was probably a driving force in the explosion of asylums, "Nervine" homes, and resting places of the 1800s. It seemed to affect women more severely than men, and physician's inability to understand the cause of suffering did nothing to increase their sympathy (or scientific inquisitiveness). They would frequently ascribe their female patient's ailments to *hysteria*, an even more humiliating diagnosis than what neurasthenia would later become.

Neurasthenia interested me not only because of the complete mystery of its origins by scientists and doctors of the day, but also because of its obvious association with mercury poisoning—something we can easily spot now, a hundred and fifty years later. As I was pouring through some of the early books on neurasthenia, looking for mention of anything resembling Alzheimer's disease or autism, this phrase caught my attention:

> *"In no complaint does it happen more frequently that the patient gets into a Vicious Circle, the fundamental disorder producing symptoms which again maintain and aggravate the disease."*[33]

I wasn't looking for autoimmunity when I read this quote, but even so, it felt like autoimmunity was somewhere in there: A disorder that produced symptoms which "again maintain and aggravate the disease" sounded similar to the concept of the body attacking itself. The body creates an improper immune response, which inadvertently creates inflammation, which creates another improper response. The "vicious circle" they were describing in neurasthenia closely resembled a component of autoimmune illness of today.

Neurasthenia described mental disorders—delirious, hysterical people with body shakes and other neurological issues. That part sounded nothing like autoimmune disorders of today, but a curious thing happened in the 1860s—Neurasthenia began to grow into something much bigger than the hysteria, fatigue and exhaustion of the earlier part of the century.

New variations appeared like *splanchnic neurasthenia*, a condition describing extreme depression and *gastric neurasthenia*, a condition dealing with frequent stomach pains and unstable bowels— descriptions which sound similar to the inflammatory bowel diseases of today. Neurasthenia would be listed as a contributing cause of *muscular rheumatism* in descriptions which echo modern day reports of rheumatoid arthritis, chronic fatigue syndrome,[34] or fibromyalgia. Weir Mitchell, a physician uniquely familiar with these issues, penned frequent neurasthenia essays touching on *causalgia*, something we might call *Complex regional pain syndrome* today.

By 1915, near the high-water mark of neurasthenia diagnoses, a book on the topic titled *The vicious circles of neurasthenia, and their treatment* would devote entire chapters to neurasthenia-caused psychoses, vascular disorders, respiratory disorders, digestive disorders, genito-urinary disorders, and even skin disorders.[35] From the period starting in the early 1800s and ending in the early 1900s, neurasthenia grew from a label assigned to those suffering purely from neurological ailments into a catch-all term that included nearly any of the newer illnesses of the day.

Perhaps a neurasthenia-related diagnosis offered comfort to those who were suffering, but in relation to understanding its origins or possible cures—it was a useless term. The doctors and scientists of 1915 had no more idea as to what was causing the spectrum of illnesses they were diagnosing than those one hundred years earlier did. Their pills and powders were similarly inadequate.

Unfortunately, this description about the understanding and treatment options for neurasthenia in 1915 may sound similar to our current state of affairs regarding autoimmune disorders. Could it be possible that all of the modern diseases we see today like Crohn's disease, Sjögren's syndrome, rheumatoid arthritis, and fibromyalgia— could all of these diseases—which scientists are still unable to explain and doctors are still unable to cure—could all of them have actually begun their abominable ascent one hundred years earlier, hidden under the veil of neurasthenia?

While the original, narrow definition of neurasthenia surfaced in various medical journals for the first half of the 1800s, its use as a diagnosis exploded after a neurologist published an article on neurasthenia in April of 1869 in the well-respected Boston Medical and Surgical Journal.[36] Why might have physicians begun to experience a need for this broader term of unexplained illness?

Just a few months later, in August, the Boston Medical and Surgical Journal would publish another article that probably had everything to do with physician's newfound need for the term. It was written by a Boston physician named Edward Wigglesworth, and he was reporting on the marvelous success he had been having with a new technique to treat syphilis which had been introduced in Europe several years earlier.[37] The drug employed was still the old standby—mercury, but the administration was decidedly new. The article was called

"Subcutaneous Injection of Corrosive Sublimate in Syphilis" and it announced the beginning of the second wave of medicinal metals. They weren't just rubs, powders or pills anymore. From now on, they could be injected.

HORROR AUTOXICUS

In the late 1800s, scientists began to realize the limitations of their most powerful microscopes. In their experiments, they would pass solutions through Chamberland filters—filters that contained holes too small for bacteria to pass through. The resulting solutions, which appeared to be free of any bacteria, even when viewed on a microscope, could still cause infections when used in additional experiments.

Louis Pasteur and other scientists of the day were confounded by this phenomenon and supposed that even though they could not see them, organisms tinier than the smallest bacteria existed and were the cause of these infections.

If you were asked to picture an image of a modern-day scientist in your mind, you would most likely think of a spectacled white-coat peering into the depths of a microscope—a Jane Goodall without the khakis—waiting for hours to capture just the right moment should it happen to appear in front of them. The reality is much more boring and tedious.

The magnification of standard optical microscopes is limited in that it relies on reflected light to project images onto the eyepiece. Most viruses are smaller than the shortest wavelength of visible light (violet[i]) and so light will never reflect off of them. Electron microscopes solved this problem and produced much higher magnifications than optical microscopes, allowing scientists to "see" viruses. But there's a problem —at these unfathomable scales, the "soup" of cells and microbes one might picture from having seen live blood cell analyses becomes a barren wasteland, where panning around the slide until a specific virus is caught becomes an art form in and of itself.

If you ever received a telescope for Christmas and discovered on the first night that its magnification was so much it was almost impossible to "find" anything in the night sky, even though you knew exactly where to aim, that is the same dilemma scientists deal with using high-powered electron microscopes. It's more difficult in the lab because the stars and planets don't stay put—they move constantly, making identification even more difficult.[ii]

The magnification isn't the problem—*locating* what you are looking for is. It is because of this that many of the scientific discoveries of the last one hundred years haven't come from one-in-a-million chance encounters caught on an electron microscope, but instead from having developed a myriad of techniques to infer what happened while they weren't looking.

It was from one of these techniques that the concept of autoimmunity first appeared. Among one of our immune system's many miracles is its stunning ability to distinguish between itself and others. In 1901, an immunologist observed that goats produced antibodies against the red blood cells of other goats, but not their own. This discovery led him to coin the phrase *horror autoxicus* – the scenario in which the body's immune system was unable to distinguish

---

i. The "v" in Roy G. Biv.
ii. Astronomers will shake their fists at my implication that the stars and planets do not move. Physicists will say it depends on your frame of reference.

between a foreign invader and itself.

Your body's immune system spends the early part of life learning the difference between foreign and self—something which explains why breastfeeding is so helpful in strengthening a baby's early immunity to disease. Getting sick is also a very good way of teaching the body what is dangerous – the "memory" of an infectious battle might still be used sixty or seventy years from now to instantly identify an old foe and quickly defeat it.

Many years after the original 1901 goat study, additional scientists began to build more evidence that horror autoxicus actually did happen. According to their research, they suggested that occasionally your body *did* appear to misidentify itself as an invader and launch a vicious attack. Despite the potential of this new line of inquiry, advances came slowly. In an era of exploding discoveries in viruses, bacteria, and the vaccines used to stop them, autoimmunity was an extremely obscure area of scientific research that few paid attention to.

Just as the concept of autoimmunity began to gain scientific interest in the 1920s, an interesting thing happened—a former topic of much discussion seemed to wane: neurasthenia, the catch-all label that had been attributed to any disorder that had no other obvious etiology or cause.

The growing field of psychiatry had undoubtedly claimed a few of the mental illnesses associated with the disease, but any mention of neurasthenia and all of its many other forms had nearly disappeared by 1930, as if a viral plague had swept through the civilized world and exhausted its supply of potential victims. Some have suggested that neurasthenia appeared to go away because it was being treated exclusively by psychiatrists who referred to it differently, but patient data from neurologists at the turn of the century indicate that 8% of their patients were still being referred to them for neurasthenia well into the 1920s.[38]

Modern reviews of neurasthenia have suggested that the disease was a cultural construct of people dealing with increased anxiety or stress—insinuating that it did not exist at all. Perhaps neurasthenia resembles autoimmune disorders more than we thought—a disease for which many people are suffering horribly and experts who can't understand its cause attribute it to a psychological origin. In retrospect, it is clear that neurasthenia and its related disorders were made possible by metals of the day—mercury and possibly lead or arsenic.

Although the era of mercury-based disease began to draw to a close by the 1950s, it is clear it will take physicians a very long time to admit the totality of this blunder. In adults and children over six-years-old, mercury-containing dental amalgams are still recommended by the FDA.[39] Mercurochrome, the mercury-containing antiseptic was never actually banned by the FDA but was re-classified as a new drug in 1998 —a classification which would require extensive testing to receive licensure, something no one has yet to undertake. And probably the most egregious vestige of medicine's two-hundred-year-old fascination with metals—a few vaccines still contain thimerosal, the mercury-based preservative. Although thimerosal began to be phased out in 1999, mercury-containing vaccines are still being injected by enlightened physicians to this day, occasionally amongst pediatric populations.

The irony of modern-day doctors laughing at the ignorance of their forefather's "blue pills" and other purgatives, while having seemingly little qualms about injecting smaller amounts of the same into their patients is lost on no one but themselves.

As Ruth Taylor, Senior Lecturer at Barts and the London School of Medicine said in her thorough evaluation of neurasthenia, "Like hysteria, there has been an apparent diminution of the prevalence of neurasthenia to the point where it actually disappeared."[40] Actually, it did not disappear. It was changing names and had only just gotten started.

METAL, MICROBES & MEDICINE

Poison, it turns out, is more easily defined by the patient than the practitioner.

This section pieces together the mechanisms that cause modern illness. While the previous section looked at medicinal metals administered between 1800-1900, this section focuses on recent scientific research—something which points to the combination of metals, microbes and medicine as a cause of man-made disease.

ALUMINUM

"It is my purpose and seems to be my duty to make these things known to the public. Apparently there is no place in America where they are taught."

—*Dr. Charles Betts*

A doctor was sick—his stomach pains had become so crippling he was told he might have only three months to live. In a last-ditch effort to save his life, he quit his practice in Ohio and moved to Colorado in search of something—anything, that might give him comfort.

He spent his days at Manitou Springs, a tiny town overlooked by Pike's Peak. Every time he filled his aluminum canteen with drinking water, he couldn't help but to notice small bubbles fizzing at the bottom. Intrigued, he noticed that someone else had a glass jar and watched as they filled water into their container. Their water was clear and motionless. No bubbles formed. No fizzing.

The doctor recalled his earlier years of chemistry, of alkalis and gases, and felt sure he understood what had been wrecking his stomach and intestines. He left the springs, returned home, and confidently discarded every aluminum container he owned. Within eight weeks, with no other changes, his health had fully returned and he was able to resume practicing medicine.

The man's name was Dr. Charles Betts. The year was 1913, and he had just realized he was experiencing what a few others had warned about—the acute toxicity of aluminum.

A controversy on the dangers of aluminum poisoning had been brewing for some time. In the 1850s, a physician from England named John Snow mapped the locations of deaths from a terrible cholera outbreak in London and determined the cause to be a contaminated water pump. Although he was ridiculed at the time, his theory would later prove correct after the water supply was cleaned up and the cholera deaths disappeared.

A little-known paper of his may come to have greater significance. In 1857, he published a report suggesting that the cause of the bone deformations—called *rickets*—children were experiencing was due to the *alum* bakers were putting in their bread. In the same way he had grasped the geographic pattern of the cholera victims, he realized that the children suffering from stunted bone growth clustered around commercial bakers who were using a new kind of baking soda containing a form of aluminum. The children whose bread was baked at home didn't seem to have any problems. Although he never pursued the contention much further, recent scientific research would seem to support his "aluminum stunts bone growth" hypothesis.[41]

Despite his warnings, aluminum was still being used in baking soda in the early 1900s. It was widely used in the manufacture of cookware and utensils and was being injected into patients before surgery, as it was thought to have coagulating effects on the blood. Most shocking of all, it was being used to clarify and purify municipal water supplies across the United States.[42]

Mercury and arsenic, long known to be toxic, didn't present the controversy that aluminum did. They had been used in medicine as purgatives and tonics. Everyone knew the chemicals were dangerous but believed they were familiar enough with the symptoms to quickly recognize any illness due to their effects. Aluminum was different. Since the late 1800s, its use had exploded in popularity as costs for its production had plummeted and no one knew for sure what its toxicological profile looked like. Regardless, this new miracle metal was being used everywhere for everything and concerns about its potential toxicity would fall on deaf ears.

In the early 1900s, a novel use for aluminum appeared by accident —as an *adjuvant* in vaccines—but unlike the cookware and water filters, there would be no readily available substitute for this one. For many years, horses were frequently used for producing large quantities of what we might now call a vaccine. They would inject an animal with a small quantity of the *Tetanus* toxoid. After a few weeks, they'd drain the horse's blood, filter out the plasma and would obtain a small amount of tetanus antitoxin they could inject into humans and hope for a protective effect. Scientists realized if they mixed a substance called *potash alum* into the tetanus toxoid, the horse might produce more than 1,000 times as much antitoxin. They didn't understand why, but there was something about the potash alum that created a very strong immune response and enabled them to multiply their output by an almost unbelievable amount.

More experiments were done over the years with different forms of aluminum and it always appeared to elevate the immune response—a phenomenon that scientists are only now beginning to understand.[43] This would become important as they strove to maximize the effectiveness of their vaccine while simultaneously using the least amount of pathogenic material to do it. There were other *adjuvants* that promoted the effectiveness of antitoxins and vaccines, but aluminum was far and away the cheapest and most powerful.

In 1921, the controversy surrounding the toxicity of aluminum was beginning to grow and a German scientist named Dollken ran some of the most thorough tests ever done to determine the true toxicity of aluminum.

> *"Like the other members of the heavy metal series aluminum therefore acts on the bowel and kidney in general poisoning, while many of the symptoms point to a direct action on the brain. Dollken has recently confirmed Siem's results, and showed that the nerve cells and fibres of the cord and medulla undergo degeneration, particularly those of the lower cranial nerves."*[44]

Even though it was discovered in 1921 that aluminum could damage cranial nerves, it's use as an adjuvant in vaccines was just beginning. As of the year 2018, over half of the vaccines children receive contain aluminum as an adjuvant. Since 1921, we've realized that cranial nerves are not the only thing that can be affected— researchers have injected aluminum hydroxide into mice and caused asthma.[45] They've rubbed aluminum hydroxide cream on the brains of monkeys and created epilepsy.[46] Many of the modern illnesses which humans now suffer from—including some autoimmune diseases—can often be recreated in laboratories with the help of aluminum adjuvants.

Numerous studies point to an unfortunate reality—aluminum is a dangerous metal to put inside the body, even in tiny amounts. It damages cells that it comes in contact with and has a particular affinity for damaging neurons—the cells inside the brain. As the corpus of scientific knowledge grows, aluminum—specifically *aluminum hydroxide*, still commonly used as a vaccine adjuvant—is being implicated in a long list of ailments and conditions, possibly more than mercury ever was. [i]

Proponents of aluminum will typically argue two points: 1) You will receive more dietary aluminum than anything you will ever be injected with. 2) There is such a tiny amount of injected aluminum that it couldn't possibly hurt anyone. Both of these stances seem perfectly reasonable, particularly upon reading the fifteen and twenty-year old scientific studies they cite. Unfortunately, more recent studies have come out in the last few years—even the last few months—that are turning everything we thought we knew about aluminum on its head.

---

i. Some people mistakenly believe that aluminum was recently placed in vaccines as a replacement for the mercury (Thimerosal) that was being removed. They serve two different purposes. Thimerosal was used as a preservative in larger, multi-dose vials that would be used many times before being discarded. Nowadays, most vaccines are produced in single-use syringes.

BB UNDER SCAR

It's a simple entry on our family calendar: "BB under scar." My wife has been thorough for all the years we've been married and has cataloged many important events on the yearly calendars that hang on our refrigerator. "Moving to LA!" and "It's a boy!" are some of the entries you will find as you flip through them. A few months after our son was born, my wife's health would take a terrifying nosedive. Entries like "Major stomach pain! Leg is killing me!" and "Brain fog! Ugg." would become more common on the calendar.

"It felt like I drank battery acid," she would tell me on our first date when she was twenty-one. She had just moved home to recover from having eighteen inches of her small intestine removed. Despite her reluctance to leave her parents' home under post-op duress, I was somehow able to talk her into a blind date.

"I crawled to the phone on my hands and knees to call 911 and wrote a goodbye note to my parents while I waited for the ambulance—everything was turning hard and shutting down."

Her small intestine had perforated, leaking stomach acid into her entire abdominal cavity, and her body was beginning to shut down. Thanks to the efforts of some extremely talented surgeons, she survived. But everything had to come out, be washed, examined, diseased parts cut out, and the remaining stitched back together. The rollercoaster ride of Crohn's would continue, complicated by scar tissue and the missing section of her intestine.

Years later, after giving birth to our son, something strange happened. Her health began to deteriorate in new ways that seemed to have nothing to do with Crohn's disease. New stomach pains that resembled nothing she had felt before. A gnawing pain high up in the stomach. A seemingly paralyzed GI tract. Crushing fatigue. Pins and needles on her face. Burning in her brain and spine. Numbness in her arm. Heart palpitations. The brain fog—that strange feeling your brain isn't working correctly but you're completely aware of it—was the scariest part.

She called me from a grocery store one day, obviously shaken.

"Can you come meet me here?" she asked, trembling. "I'm at the Six Points grocery store."

"What's wrong?" I asked, confident I was prepared for the worst.

"I don't know," she said. "I bought groceries, and when I was checking out, I forgot my pin number. And then I couldn't sign my name. I couldn't remember my signature."

My hands began to shake—rivers of adrenaline coursed through my body. This was an entirely new level of worry. Her gut was a crotchety old friend that had its quirks—she could deal with it, as much of a pain as it was. But forgetting your own signature, that thing you probably do multiple times a day, every day of your adult life—it was obvious that something was seriously wrong.

It wouldn't be until many years later, as some of the research I had been doing began to come together, that we would go back through each and every entry on the family calendars in an attempt try to piece together what might have happened. As we worked our way backwards through some of the most horrible days and weeks, we passed the grocery store episode and saw a strange item on the calendar.

"BB under scar," the entry read.

"What was that?" I asked.

"Don't you remember?" she asked me. "That little BB? That round knot I got under my scar?"

She pointed to her abdomen, where the section of small intestine had been removed, and I remembered exactly what she was talking about. Years ago, she had me roll my finger over her scar and directly underneath was a hard ball that felt about the size of a BB from an air gun. You could move it a bit from side to side, but it was an unmistakable mass.

"Never been there before?" I asked.

"Never," she said, and I believed her. She logged every little detail with her health.

I skimmed back through the calendar and saw something that both of us had completely forgotten about. A tiny event with a not-so-tiny result. The details came flooding back in a flash.

"New patient appointment at family doctor—TDaP," the entry read. Instantly, we knew what had happened to her.

GRANULOMAS

In the 1990s, scientists began to hear of a new disease that was appearing throughout France—adults were complaining of severe shoulder pain accompanied by disabling chronic fatigue and memory loss. Doctors had no idea what might be causing it and the scientists were stumped as well. Biopsies from their deltoid muscle, the frequent site of pain, revealed lesions that contained mostly macrophages— white blood cells. Inside the white blood cells was an unidentified substance comprised of nanocrystals. Further research identified what the substance was—aluminum hydroxide, the adjuvant used in vaccines.

What had happened to cause this sudden outbreak of a seemingly new disorder? It would turn out a large campaign by the French health department had been launched to persuade adults to receive a new Hepatitis B vaccine. Simultaneously, the recommended vaccine administration site was changed from subcutaneous, just below the skin, to intramuscular, which is deep within the muscle. These two changes converged to create such a huge spike in peculiar symptoms it was obvious there was a serious problem that needed investigation. They would term the illness *macrophagic myofasciitis*[47] (MMF), meaning inflammation of the muscle due to white blood cells.

Some of the granulomas were found at injection sites that were 10 years old.[48] And shockingly the aluminum was still contained inside and perfectly preserved. Unsurprisingly, many in the scientific community deny aluminum had anything to do with these people's symptoms. Another similar event happened a few years later that would make this denial very difficult.

In 1998, an insect-borne infection called "Bluetongue" returned to Europe after having been absent for 50 years. The virus infected sheep and prevented those who survived from being commercially available for sale or export. Within ten years, the virus had spread and the European Union decided to vaccinate all sheep and lambs within Europe against the disease. There are two different vaccines available for the Bluetongue virus and the sheep received two courses of each. Within thirty days, the sheep had received 16 milligrams[i] of aluminum.

Over the course of the next few months, these sheep began to experience a new disorder that veterinarians had never seen. They began to lose weight and experience neurological problems. Later they would show signs of extreme fatigue, paralysis, then death. The sheep were autopsied and the cause for their paralysis was clear—lesions on their spinal cords—lesions that contained aluminum.[49]

Concerned that the recent vaccination program was killing the sheep, researchers decided to do an experiment to see if they could track the path of the aluminum. Vaccine makers have routinely claimed that although the aluminum their products contain may be dangerous, it is excreted from the body within a few weeks of injection and will pose no harm afterwards.

The study followed three flocks of twenty-six sheep. Over the

---

i. Yes, milligrams.

course of fifteen months, one group received the routine schedule of 19 vaccine injections (which also contained aluminum). The second flock received the same shots containing the same amount of aluminum administered to the first group but without the antigen contained in the vaccines. The third group received a saline placebo.[50]

When the study was over, they began looking at the skin of the sheep where they had been injected and were disturbed by what they found. Unsurprisingly, the saline placebo group had no issues. But the other two groups had developed granulomas at the injection site—fibrous tissue created by the body in an attempt to wall off a foreign invader.

In some animals, they were able to recover one granuloma per vaccine. The sheep had created protective tissue around the ingredients of each injection in order to protect themselves from the contents and amazingly, the granulomas were still there—at least fifteen months later.

They biopsied the granulomas and discovered them teeming with white blood cells, still active and full of aluminum. Obviously concerned, they were curious if the aluminum could move further than just the subcutaneous granulomas and took a look at some of the sheep's lymph nodes and spinal tissue.

Both areas of the sheep—the lymph nodes and spinal column—contained the same aluminum-filled white blood cells as the subcutaneous granulomas. The aluminum had been transported, deep into the body. The results of this study should be concerning to anyone who has ever been injected with aluminum. While the subcutaneous granulomas of aluminum might be disturbing, the sheep with *more* granulomas may have had less aluminum in their spinal cord and lymph nodes. The granulomas may have done their job and protected the sheep from further harm.

With macrophages myofasciitis, they had seen symptoms of disease and examined what they could via biopsy. The dots connected, but they couldn't conduct autopsies on living patients, and they could not attempt to replicate the scenario on human subjects. The sheep presented a unique opportunity that had never been conducted in studies of aluminum toxicity. They were able to spot a new disease that had never appeared amongst sheep, come up with a reason for it, then replicate the origin of the disease under the exact conditions which they suspected caused it in the first place.

The research was now clear—the aluminum had caused the mysterious new disease, but that wasn't the most disturbing part. The aluminum from vaccines was not being excreted from the body in two or three weeks. Not fifteen months, and not even ten years in some cases, as was seen in some of the MMF research. Some of the aluminum might go on to harm immediately after the injection, but the rest of it might be safely tucked away around the body in granulomas—a collection of deadly time-release capsules—waiting to erupt.

THE WAY IT MOVES

Although humans ingest a small amount of aluminum in their diet, only about .3% of it is actually absorbed into the body. Ingested aluminum is in an ionic form that is easily filtered by the kidneys and can be stopped from causing neurological damage by the blood brain barrier. The aluminum that is injected is in a different form called nanoparticulates. This form of aluminum is much different than the ingested kind and creates a couple of problems you will never see with the dietary kind.

If you were to take the aluminum contained in a single pediatric vaccine and inject it into a specific part of a child's brain, possibly the *pineal gland* or the *area postrema*, they would almost certainly die. The amount of aluminum hydroxide in many of the shots children regularly receive is toxic enough to kill anyone if it was administered directly into the wrong spot.

The safety in injected aluminum has always been in its dilution. The dose is deadly—we know that—but it was assumed it was distributed around the body. If not evenly, then at least spread out in some way so as to minimize the chance of it ending up in one specific place where it might cause serious problems.

Until recently, we made the logical assumption that the less aluminum the vaccine contained, the less of it might make it into dangerous areas of your body—a perfectly reasonable notion. We depended on that inference to assuage our fears of serious harm from the ingredients in vaccines. If the amount of aluminum contained in the vaccine was so little, then the chance of a significant portion of the metal reaching your brain would be infinitesimally small.

An astonishing discovery about aluminum was made recently—less aluminum is worse. Less aluminum is *more* dangerous.[51] In the study, researchers injected mice with varying amounts of aluminum and looked at three factors: their behavior, markers for immune system activation in the brain, and actual amounts of the metal in their brain. Across the study, mice who received less aluminum per injection fared worse—their behaviors indicated neurological abnormalities and the amount of aluminum that reached their brain was much higher. The two higher dosages of aluminum seemed to have insignificant effects.

How could this be? When a vaccine is injected into your arm, the aluminum triggers an aggressive immune response and your body begins to mount an attack against it. This is often why your arm gets so sore after a vaccine—it's your body forming granulomas around the aluminum—a collection of immune cells doing their best to wall off the invader.

Scientists now understand that your body responds more aggressively with granuloma formations at higher concentrations of aluminum. It makes sense when you think about it—the more dangerous the invader is perceived to be, the more aggressive the attack becomes. If you get a large dose of aluminum, the body works hard to wall it off inside protective granulomas. But the opposite scenario is more concerning – if the injection contains a smaller amount of aluminum, *more* of it makes it into your lymphatic system and bloodstream because there is less granuloma formation. This stunning realization should change the entire way we calculate safe levels of exposure to metal, especially in regard to aluminum.

Another mystery has been solved about how aluminum travels. If you were to have a small amount of aluminum in your body, you might imagine it floating around freely, possibly causing a tiny bit of damage if it were to land in a vulnerable area. Studies have recently shed light on how nanoparticulate aluminum moves throughout your body—it's not random at all, but within the white blood cells themselves.[52]

When a metal like aluminum is injected into your body, your immune system's white blood cells attempt to destroy it.[53] But they can't destroy it, because it's a metal—so the aluminum just sits inside the white blood cell until it dies, at which point the metal is immediately picked up by another white blood cell. Even inside granulomas this recycling process takes place over and over.

Because aluminum moves around your body within white blood cells, this presents a very big problem. White blood cells are the frontline defense of your immune system, and they go where they are signaled to help. Your immune system employs a sophisticated communication network, creating proteins like *MCP-1* to alert the immune system where help is needed. If you have a cut on your leg, your body will send out signals asking for white blood cells to go to that area. If you have an ulcer in your stomach, your body will ask for help there.

Your body is very complex, and even makes predictions about where help might be needed. A 2009 study has profound implications for how metal may get signaled to the brain. Through their research, scientists found that blocking the bile ducts on rats caused their brain to create MCP-1 and signal for help[54] from the immune system. Even though the inflammation was in their liver, their brain was asking for help. We can only guess what purpose this signaling fulfills, but the realization that inflammation anywhere in the body might summon white blood cells to the brain foreshadows much about how aluminum is causing so much neurological damage.

In addition to understanding that aluminum is transported around your body via white blood cells, this signaling concept is one of the most important things to remember: Metal goes where the inflammation is. It hijacks your body's immune response by hitching a ride within the white blood cells that respond to the call for help.

Another safety net we thought would protect us from metal toxicity is a defensive shield called the *blood brain barrier*. It's an additional layer of protection around sensitive parts of the brain to prevent anything dangerous from getting inside—an important defense mechanism considering how crucial the brain's functions are to life.

Many people picture the blood brain barrier as a balloon around the outside of the brain—a thin membrane that encapsulates the brain itself. It's actually a secondary coating around the thousands and thousands of blood vessels within the brain. Blood vessels elsewhere in the body are purposefully leaky so that plasma can escape into surrounding tissue and get recycled into the lymphatic system—a process by which your immune system can identify pathogens in your blood.

But in parts of the brain protected by this barrier, the blood vessels have an extra layer around them to prevent this exchange from happening. Some parts of your brain such as the *area postrema* do not have this layer of protection by design—the area postrema is responsible for triggering nausea and vomiting and needs a clear picture of the toxins present in your body.

White blood cells can freely pass through the blood brain barrier and unfortunately, many of these white blood cells may contain aluminum inside. In the past, discussions were had about the timing of the formation of the blood brain barrier in neonates and the lack of protection their brain had from invaders. Now that we've discovered aluminum is being transported within the white blood cells, the blood brain barrier suddenly becomes a trivial component—when hidden inside the white blood cells, the aluminum will pass right through.

The realization that aluminum does not leave your body quickly at all, but could possibly stay there for years is very concerning. Remember that aluminum is placed in vaccines specifically to cause an exaggerated immune response to the pathogens they contain. Unfortunately, aluminum has no prejudice and can create a heightened response to nearly anything—from peanuts to surgical titanium screws to silicone implants.

Injected aluminum creates problems in the body—it is a neurotoxin and readily damages tissue. It remains in the body for years, possibly decades. While these traits of aluminum are extremely troubling, there is one more feature that may eclipse them all.

INTRACELLULAR BACTERIA

We know that metal can travel around the body via white blood cells. We know that immune activation events signal for help from white blood cells—many of which may contain metal. It's fairly obvious that when areas of your body are signaling for help but inadvertently get a toxin like aluminum, bad things can happen. There is a third factor that may impact the course of illness as much, if not more, than these other two, and to understand that, we need to talk about microbes for a moment.

Viruses are interesting creatures, if you can call them that. They aren't "living" in the traditional sense. For one thing, they can't reproduce on their own. They depend on being able to multiply inside living cells. Bacteria aren't like this—they can replicate on their own. Many years ago, a microbiologist named Emmy Klieneberger-Nobel discovered a new type of bacteria. These special bacteria, which could reproduce normally, could also lose their cell wall, enter inside another cell, and reproduce like viruses.ⁱ. Some bacteria, which had always been thought of as reproducing differently from viruses, could apparently do the same thing. When they lost their cell wall, they could sneak inside another cell, reproduce, then exit the cell and change back into their original version.

This trick allows these stealthy pathogens to proliferate where other bacteria can't, creating a trail of inflammation that is difficult to spot. Why? Intracellular bacteria are very difficult to see on a microscope—they don't look like normal bacteria because they don't have an easily detectable cell wall. They're also inside other cells for much of their life cycle, camouflaging their presence even further. Lastly, staining techniques that allow researchers to more readily identify normal bacteria can fail on these intracellular parasites. Even *polymerase chain reaction* (PCR)—one of the most sensitive techniques for detecting DNA fragments—can have a difficult time finding them.

Because of this, people may experience the inflammation from cell wall deficient bacteria, but even a skilled researcher with expensive tools would have a difficult time detecting them. As scientists try to understand the nature of autoimmune disease and continually describe the immune system as attacking "itself," it begs the question if perhaps your immune system is actually attacking something it can detect is there—but something we cannot easily see?

Intracellular bacteria have another trait that makes them even more dangerous—they have an affinity for macrophages, a type of white blood cell. Once the bacteria lose their cell wall, they will sneak inside your white blood cells to reproduce, presumably rendering the unfortunate white blood cells unable to function.

This presents a problem—a "vicious circle." These bacteria are naturally going to create inflammation, something we experience as the

---

i. Also called L-form bacteria, intracellular bacteria, and cell wall deficient forms. These are all essentially the same thing.

symptoms of being sick – fever, pain, fatigue, soreness, etc. But the white blood cells that arrive to help become unwitting incubators for more bacteria—which creates more inflammation—which calls for more white blood cells… And so on, and so on. In this scenario, your immune system is constantly trying to get the upper hand, but cannot.

In all of human history, chronic inflammation had never been a problem. You might get extremely sick from a virus or a bacteria, but you would either live or die—one of those two things. If you died, well then, that was not a good thing. If you lived, you would have permanent immunity to that which had infected you. Your body might have horrible scars to show for it, but you would have won the battle, fair and square, never to be bothered again by that particular invader. This harsh microbial reality governed human's existence for all of time —until recently.

What changed? If these intracellular bacteria create the vicious circle that leads to chronic inflammation, why weren't they a problem for all of human history?

The concept of bacteria losing their cell wall and replicating inside your white blood cells—this is not a normal lifecycle for bacteria. It may have been happening for millions of years, but if so, it was a very rare occurrence. As it turns out, a couple of relatively modern inventions cause bacteria to lose their cell walls and have made what used to be an extremely rare circumstance far too common.

We are still learning what things have this effect on certain bacteria, but three things that we know promote this effect are irradiating food, microwaves and pasteurized milk. Commercial vendors will often use ionizing radiation or pasteurization to kill viruses and bacteria in food or milk to lessen the risk of disease. When you microwave your food, which is a different process than irradiation, a similar effect happens— bacteria inside the food can lose their cell wall.[55] If the bacteria in the food are not killed, but have lost their cell wall, this can promote their ability to proliferate once they are in the presence of macrophages.

Although the food and milk we consume can contain cell wall deficient bacteria, I believe this is unlikely to be the cause of chronic inflammation. It certainly doesn't help, but it's unlikely to cause the long-running infections we see today. For one, I don't think the numbers of intracellular bacteria are likely to be high enough to work in their favor. Secondly, I think the thing that causes the destruction of the bacterial cell walls needs to be inside your body.

Because these things *induce* the bacteria to lose their cell wall, I will refer to them as *inductors*. Before inductors existed, your immune system could easily gain the upper hand and kill off bacterial infections. Ever since humans began using these inductors, the back-and-forth struggle for survival of these microbes in our body become a months-long, sometimes years-long affair. What would have once been settled in days or weeks might now go on seemingly forever. This change, from normal bacteria to ones without cell walls might seem a trivial change, but it tipped the scales in favor of these intracellular creatures.

One of the most common inductors that nearly everyone has consumed are *antibiotics*. Antibiotics are very good inductors because they're designed to strip the cell wall from the bacteria. In fact, it's common practice in laboratories to use penicillin *purposefully* to transform some types of bacteria so their intracellular forms can be studied. For many bacteria, this process will kill them, but for those it doesn't, they may lose their cell wall and become intracellular. For these bacteria, stripping their cell wall actually *encourages* their reproduction and proliferation.

The *penicillin* family of antibiotics can be particularly problematic. For some bacteria, such as the *Streptococcus* family, they often thrive specifically because of their interaction with certain antibiotics. I have seen Strep infections treated with one of the penicillin family of antibiotics grow all the way from the throat until it becomes a *perianal strep* (rectal strep) infection. These poor kids will receive course after course of antibiotic with no apparent effect other than perhaps a change in the location of the infection. I've seen a kid with a strep infection treated with amoxicillin, only to have what appeared to be Crohn's disease in his terminal ileum a few weeks later.[ii]

Allergic to penicillin?

Some people will claim to be allergic to penicillin or one of several other antibiotics. While this phenomenon does appear to exist, for most people what they experienced wasn't an allergic reaction at all, but possibly the immune system reacting to an explosion of growth of intracellular bacteria.

Mothers have noticed their children break out in hives after an antibiotic, an event so frequent it has a name—amoxicillin rash. Unless this is something that happens within an hour or two of receiving the antibiotic, it's probably not allergy. If your child happens to have the right bacteria in their body, the antibiotic can create the perfect breeding ground for its growth and inadvertently cause a massive infection that may be unrelated to their initial problem. The rashes on your child's back or legs or arms may be their body trying to deal with that infection. It seems that many doctors and nurses aren't familiar with this concept and will say your child has an allergy to the antibiotic. It may not be an allergy, but a bacterial infection that's been unleashed. The bacteria has lost its cell wall, invaded white blood cells, and has now turned from an acute infection to a chronic one, hiding inside the cells of the immune system—inside the cells that were supposed to kill it.

Other bacteria are known to exhibit these effects such as *C.*

---

ii. Please see the chapter on Crohn's and ulcerative colitis for more discussion of this topic.

pneumoniae and *Mycobacterium*. Because this is such a poorly understood subject, a complete list may be impossible to determine. I believe many other bacteria, possibly all of them, can shed their cell wall and reproduce in other macrophages under the right conditions.[56] Pure speculation, but you will occasionally see events that would seem to support this notion. Even though viruses reproduce inside other cells, there appears to be some evidence that viruses and antibiotics together can accelerate bacterial growth, as evidenced by the fact that patients with mononucleosis infections (Epstein-Barre virus) often develop large rashes following a course of amoxicillin.[57] Perhaps the immune system is already devoting large numbers of white blood cells to fight the viral infection and the additional immunological load of intracellular bacteria becomes too much.

A more complete list of problematic and recommended antibiotics is listed in the Healing and Recovery section. Keep these potential issues with antibiotics in mind if you or someone you know has taken them and began to experience chronic inflammation. As we move forward in learning about the nature of chronic illness, it's important to understand how antibiotics can unwillingly contribute to the problem. But there's one more inductor that I think trumps them all— aluminum.

METALS, MICROBES & MEDICINE

As I studied the toxicity of aluminum and realized how it could easily be transported around the body to areas of inflammation, my wife kept insisting there were microbes involved. She had studied cell wall deficient forms for many years as she tried to understand what might be causing her health issues, and was convinced there was a microbial component to what she was suffering from. She did suspect however, that mercury—from fillings as a child and adult—was a key player in why her immune system was not able to prevail over intracellular bacteria and other infections.

I thought Crohn's might be due purely to aluminum toxicity, but realized there were many features of the disease that didn't sit well with that notion: The way it could spread. The way it could go away for months, even years at a time, only to return with a vengeance with no apparent reason. There were other strange illnesses that struck me— particularly systemic things like full body rashes. I couldn't understand how aluminum alone could trigger disruptions in the skin all over someone's body—aluminum doesn't appear to circulate in the blood or lymph for long, but comes to rest in granulomas, muscle tissue and organs.

As we discussed the nature of autoimmune disease and chronic illness, a thought occurred to her: If antibiotics could induce classic bacteria into cell wall deficient forms, allowing them to evade the immune system, avoid detection, to reproduce, and cause chronic inflammation, perhaps aluminum could too. Perhaps aluminum could turn an innocuous bacteria into a long running sickness, even sustaining the infection by keeping the white blood cells from being able to function and eradicate the infection. And maybe it could create an even more comfortable environment for the intracellular bacteria to thrive.

This wasn't a thought out of left field, and appears to be supported by scientific research. I had been zeroing in on the role of aluminum in man-made disease at the same time she was circling around the microbial component. Our research paths would occasionally cross but never truly aligned until we found a 2007 paper out of the Carmel Medical Center in Israel titled "Aluminum is a Potential Environmental Factor for Crohn's Disease Induction." Although it didn't complete the circle, the paper made it clear how both aluminum and certain bacteria might contribute to Crohn's disease. We had spent years on separate paths, but the intersection of metal and microbe became evident—a possible explanation for Crohn's, obvious:

"Once the aluminum-loaded organism is incorporated into the host, Aluminum enhances the organism's ability to induce a prominent granulomatous immune response, this giving rise to the pathologic features of CD."[58]

It was refreshing and exciting to see we weren't the only ones who had considered the relationship between metal and microbe as the cause of chronic disease, and especially Crohn's Disease.

Although more studies are needed to understand it completely, aluminum appears to affect cell wall integrity.[59] We know that part of aluminum's toxicity is in its ability to bind to cell membranes[60] and some believe this exact mechanism might be why it's so neurotoxic.

In fact, this ability may be part of the reason it's such a necessary ingredient in vaccines. Without the aluminum, many vaccines would not work at all. Because their components have been so weakened, they do not invoke an immune response. When you add aluminum, your response is much stronger. What causes this is poorly understood, even one hundred years after its effect was first discovered.

It's possible that aluminum's ability to affect the cell walls of bacteria may be the very reason it works as an adjuvant in vaccines. Think of the story of how aluminum's properties were first discovered—it was injected into horses alongside the tetanus toxoid. Without the aluminum, the horse would only create a small amount of antitoxin, but *with* the aluminum, it would create far more. They didn't know why, but perhaps the reason is the way in which aluminum creates intracellular versions of bacteria, giving them the unnatural ability to thrive, hide and proliferate.[i]

Put another way, an injection of tetanus bacteria alone might create a tiny battle which your body's immune system could easily win. With the intracellular boost from aluminum, the bacteria might become much more powerful, able to avoid detection, growing in number and destroying white blood cells along the way. Your body may still emerge victorious, but rather than the little skirmish it had without the aluminum, it would have fought an epic war—the evidence clearly visible by the massive amount of antibodies your immune system produced in order to win.

This may explain why aluminum is often described as *protracting*

---

i. The tetanus toxoid was not supposed to contain *Clostridium tetani*, the bacteria responsible for tetanus infections, but a purified form of *Tetanospasmin*, a neurotoxin that bacteria produced.

the immune response. It's simply giving certain bacteria a significant advantage in providing for their proliferation—something which might turn a twenty-four-hour affair into weeks of effort. Perhaps we should change our definition of aluminum adjuvant from "increases the immune response" to "*prolongs* the immune response." This seemingly trivial difference may explain much.

If aluminum *is* an inductor and can create intracellular bacteria like certain antibiotics can, the mechanism for many of our modern diseases becomes obvious.

Metals like aluminum are neurotoxins. If they get in the brain or nervous system tissue, they can destroy. Metals can also cause inflammation in other parts of the body. Aluminum is known to increase the body's immune response to pathogens, and that may be because of its ability to strip the wall from bacteria, providing a way for them to become chronic infections.

If you have metals in your body, and something triggers your immune system to signal for help, it will inadvertently draw metals to that location. Metals and antibiotics in your body can cause what would have been a simple, localized bacterial infection to become systemic and prolonged.

I believe this sequence may be the reason for *chronic* inflammation —an phenomenon associated with inflammatory bowel disease, lupus, rheumatoid arthritis, multiple sclerosis, sarcoidosis and many other illnesses. Although it may seem unlikely, I believe it may explain how this chain of events may also be responsible for neurological diseases like Alzheimer's, Parkinson's, multiple sclerosis and ALS. Heart disease. Some cancers. Anemia. Even Zika, the mosquito-borne illness that was here and gone in 2015.

As we continue on this journey to understand the nature of modern disease, keep these three concepts in mind: Metals like aluminum can travel around the body inside white blood cells. Immune activation events signal for help from these white blood cells in particular areas. Inductors like antibiotics and aluminum may be able to cause (and sustain) chronic inflammation through the creation of intracellular bacteria. A combination of these three concepts might be the cause for nearly all man-made disease.

TRIGGERED

Another thing I had noticed were patterns in the onset of disease. Having researched for years into my wife's conditions—and hearing from others who had suffered—the patterns were obvious: the beginning of nearly all the modern diseases always happened after a significant event. Through logging many stories of illness—Crohn's, autism, multiple sclerosis, chronic fatigue, Parkinson's, lupus, rheumatoid arthritis, Hashimoto's—I was able to catalog their onset and discovered four main *triggers*: An infection, pregnancy, extreme physical exertion or stress. There were a few others like surgery or seasonal changes, but it was apparent something was causing these diseases to happen. The people that were silently suffering so much could nearly always point to something very specific that triggered the onset—it wasn't a slow fade, but a particular life event—an entry on their refrigerator calendar. The connection may have not made sense, but it was there.

"I was diagnosed with rheumatoid arthritis after my first pregnancy," I would hear again and again.

"I started college and was diagnosed with Crohn's my freshman year," another refrain.

"I began training for my first marathon and developed Chronic Fatigue or Fibromyalgia, not sure which, within a few months."

Stories like these bounced around my head as I tried to connect them together. The triggers were nearly always the same: infection, pregnancy, extreme physical exertion or stress. It didn't make sense until I heard a story from a friend who was trying to understand something strange that had happened to her—a story I quickly realized was all too familiar.

"I've never felt that terrible," she said. "I'd been swimming for an hour or two and I had to get out because I couldn't move. It was like I suddenly had the flu without the fever. I was so tired I could barely make it back up onto the beach."

I instantly noted the exertion trigger and asked her about any previous medical conditions.

"Had you been sick or diagnosed with anything recently?"

"No," she said. "I had gone to the doctor a few weeks earlier, but that was just to get a tetanus shot after I stepped on something at the farm."

"And you hadn't felt bad since then?"

"No, not really. My arm was hard as a rock, but they said it might be. I mean, I wasn't feeling great, but nothing I would have gone to the doctor for."

I looked at my wife, who had also mysteriously developed an intense, full-body fatigue soon after a TDaP shot.

"There was one thing," our friend said, "something strange. I had this lump under my scar."

She pointed at her neck where a mark from thyroid surgery was barely visible.

"It had never been there before, and suddenly this little lump appeared under my scar. Know what that might be?"

My wife and I looked at each other in amazement. It was just like her "BB." Under the scar tissue from surgery, and just after a TDaP shot —a granuloma had formed, seemingly out of thin air. That tiny little detail—so seemingly insignificant she had almost forgotten about it— was a huge clue for me.

When you get a cut on your skin, it's not just blind luck that a couple of white blood cells happen to pass by to fight off infection— your body actively signals for help from that area. White blood cells answer the call and make sure that nothing nasty gets too far into your body to harm you.

The immune system is said to be the least understood component of the human body—the last frontier in understanding. Even the brain is thought by some to hold fewer mysteries than the immune system. One of the things that is being studied intensely are the immune system's signaling mechanisms. Which signaling proteins are generated when? And from where? Who responds to them? What shuts them off? How do they know where to go based on these proteins? How do other events positively and negatively affect these signaling mechanisms? It's a secret communication network that exists within your body just now coming to light—a miracle of complexity that silently directs your body's healing mechanisms anywhere they are needed.

Something that has long been clear—these signaling mechanisms are triggered by what are called *immune activation events*. Anytime your immune system is triggered, this event initiates signaling mechanisms that your body responds to. The primary response for this request is to send white blood cells to the area signaling for help. But unfortunately in this modern age—with a very nasty material occupying many of our white blood cells—help is not what they bring.

TRIGGERS & EXERTION

After seeing two people report lumps under scar tissue after the aluminum-containing tetanus shot, I could guess that amongst the white blood cells floating around in their blood and lymph, some of them had inadvertently picked up recently injected aluminum before being summoned to the scar tissue. This was surprising to me on two accounts. It suggested that scar tissue—even though it was many years old and perfectly healed—was still causing inflammation and immune signaling. Secondly, I was surprised that a single TDaP shot, though it contained just under .4 milligrams of aluminum, might generate a such a large granuloma—an easily detectable lump at the site of inflammation.

Something occurred to me—the first of many terrifying thoughts I would have as I began to unravel this mystery. All of the recommendations regarding metal toxicity—in particular mercury and aluminum—were generated with a very common-sense assumption. When you pour a packet of Kool-Aid flavored mix into a jar of water, it spreads into the water and without much stirring, will evenly disperse into a uniform concentration. It was assumed that metals behaved similarly. If you inject .4 milligrams of aluminum into the body, it will spread out and disperse evenly into a concentration that shouldn't be remotely harmful. Over time (over a *very* long time as would later turn out) your body could excrete the metal.

It was becoming clear to me the aluminum didn't disperse evenly in your body like flavored drink powder but was aggregating and traveling to areas of inflammation—places of weakness in the body. In what seemed like a coordinated attack, it was hijacking the body's main system of defense and riding alongside to target areas of the body that were are already vulnerable—places that were signaling for help via immune activation events. The horror of how this metal was capable of so much damage was only just beginning to become evident.

After cycling through the different disease onset triggers I had noticed, it became obvious they were all immune activation events. Infection—immune activation event. Pregnancy—immune activation event. Exertion—immune activation. Stress—immune activation. They all created scenarios in which massive amounts of white blood cells were potentially being signaled for help—but instead of help, they brought highly toxic aluminum. A payload of destruction, delivered to the most vulnerable areas of your body, with the precision a modern physician could only dream of.

The signaling was poorly understood, for certain, but there were many illnesses that began to make sense to me, particularly in light of the triggers that were attributed to their onset. Like a sequence of falling dominos, many of the diseases I had been chasing around for years with nothing to show began to make sense. Plausible explanations as to why these mysterious diseases began out of nowhere—and just as importantly, why they could not be explicitly diagnosed or healed by current medical models.

* * *

Physical Exertion

Whenever you hear a story of a young person being affected with heart disease, such as myocarditis, you often will hear the confused reactions of their friends and family regarding how athletic or in-shape that person was: "They ran 5 miles every day," or "they were constantly at the gym."

It is uncommon to see an obese, 24-year-old smoker die from heart disease. Despite those two very common risk factors, it seems like it is the physically fit who often suffer more. Perhaps the news prefers to cover these sensational stories of healthy, beautiful people struck down in their prime, but regardless, indiscriminate attacks of illness often seem to affect those who ought to be immune.

There are quite a few modern diseases which people attribute their onset to exertion or exercise. I have heard many stories of women starting college, taking up an aggressive exercise regimen to stave off the dreaded "freshman 15" weight gain, only to develop ulcerative colitis or fibromyalgia. A lot of the girls with devastating side effects from the Gardasil vaccine were basketball players, volleyball players and dancers—a pattern noticed by many others.

Even FDR, the former U.S. president who was stricken with polio at 39, spent the day before his paralysis swimming with his children and running through the woods near their summer home. Exertion would become so tightly entwined with polio that posters hung in every school and doctor's office would warn children to "Not get overtired." I think there are a couple of reasons you see this connection time and again and they're not going to comfort any of you who are athletic.

There are two reasons I believe that extreme physical exertion is attributed to the onset of illness, and the first is inflammation. Extreme physical activity is always going to cause inflammation in your body, be it your joints or muscles. We know that inflammation causes your body to send white blood cells to help, and in many cases the white blood cells will contain metal.

I don't think it's any accident that cardio-heavy athletes can frequently be the ones who suffer from diseases of the heart. In a natural world, their exercise would build healthy muscle tissue. In a body that is suffering the chronic inflammation of a bacterial infection such as *Streptococcus pyogenes*, this inflammation only serves to further the damage the bacteria may be causing. As the body attempts to repair damaged muscle tissue, the inflammation may result in the abnormal cell growth seen in the "Giant Cell" diseases.

I have heard of a few cases of post-Gardasil paralysis where the damage seems to mirror the location of inflammation caused by the sport that person was active in. Because we know that white blood cells go to where they are signaled in the human body, it only makes sense that areas of inflammation would receive the brunt of metal toxicity.

The second reason I believe exertion is commonly associated with the onset of modern illness is a very simple concept, one that is actually supported by another trigger I've seen mentioned in much of the older medical literature: temperature changes. Although season and winter triggers have a separate immunological concept to them, they also create a scenario in which someone gets very warm from exertion, then gets very cold.

Cases like this appear through the medical literature. In the account of the first polio outbreak in the United States in 1894 Vermont, it was noted "The immediate apparent cause is stated in 37 instances. Of these overheating is mentioned 24 times, chilling of the body 4 times…"[61]

What's happening? The granulomas are breaking down. The fibrous collections of white blood cells that are stored around your body are being ruptured by heavy, physical exertion, releasing the aluminum into your lymphatic and circulatory systems. We know that granulomas form as a response to aluminum being injected into your body. We also know that they can stay there as along as ten years, possibly more. We can assume that the granulomas will eventually break down, releasing their contents into the body.

Perhaps this would explain why sweating is known to be an excretory route for aluminum.[62] Heat has been shown to inhibit granuloma formation.[63] I am guessing the physical torsion of heavy exertion combined with the heat it produces is disrupting some of the granulomas tucked away in your body and releasing a small load of aluminum. Although we know that some granulomas form in the skin, there are possibly less obvious ones that form deep within the muscle tissue. Many of the old medical cases often mention people "foolishly" exposing themselves to cold after being hot from exertion. Perhaps the shivering from this sequence of events—even the mere act of being cold during the winter—works in such a way as to encourage the release of metal from the granulomas within the muscle tissue.

The body's ability to form and maintain the integrity of these granulomas may be one of the biggest indicators as to who will suffer the effects from aluminum toxicity. If your body aggressively forms granulomas and something were to happen later to disrupt them, that aluminum might have the opportunity to travel to places where it could cause serious damage.

This concept will play a very big part as we learn how to heal from metal toxicity. If chelating agents designed to remove metal from your body cannot penetrate these granulomas, they may be leaving much behind. This is not a comforting thought but needs to be taken into account as we advance our knowledge of metal chelation.

There is a distinct connection between physical exertion and the onset of many of these modern diseases. It is such a frequently occurring association that it would be difficult to believe it is coincidence. Whether it is purely from inflammation, or possibly from triggering the inadvertent release of stored metal, physical exercise— once the domain of good health—may have become a risky endeavor.

STRESS, PREGNANCY & SEASONAL CHANGES

Stress can activate the immune system in ways that are impossible for any of the other triggers mentioned. In particular, the stress from not being able to respond to a fight or flight threat seems to create particularly devastating effects. In a study on rats with an artificially-induced autoimmune disease, researchers were able to make their symptoms worse simply by denying them the ability to respond to a perceived threat.[64] Similarly, a particular type of New World monkey will routinely develop the symptoms of ulcerative colitis and even colon cancer simply by being captured and caged.[65] Even in cancer studies, a common trait of those who were stricken is repressed anger—the inability to express a strong emotion. A "helplessness-prone personality" alone was used to predict cancer rates in women who had abnormal Pap smears with up to a 75% accuracy.[66]

The chemical effects of stress will also show up in your gut. It has been said that over 70% of your immune system resides in your intestines. Food digestion also requires a significant amount of energy and when the energy normally allocated for maintaining a healthy gut is sent elsewhere, bowel problems—in the form of constipation or diarrhea—will often follow.

The consequences of stress—particularly through immobilization and restraint (discussed in more detail in the autism chapters)—can trigger the immune system in deleterious ways that no change in food or exercise regimen could touch. And while extreme physical exertion may only be possible for a few hours, and pregnancy will only last for a few months, stress can exist for years—even decades—wearing down the immune system to nearly nothing.

Pregnancy

When you become pregnant, your body begins a very complex sequence of events that prepare for the creation of new life. For years it was thought the basic effect of pregnancy was the "down-regulation" of the immune system.[67] Why? Because you are growing new tissue inside you, your body might have the tendency to reject it—almost like it would a tumor. To prevent this, it was thought portions of your immune system were turned off to prevent your body from thinking of the fetus as an invader.

This seems to make sense but begs the question—wouldn't a growing baby be uniquely susceptible to the inflammation from infection? Why would the body work in such a way to maximize the chance a fetus would suffer from the effects of the mother's cold or fever? As it turns out, the immunological alterations that happen during pregnancy are much more complex than we realized—it is not a complete down-regulation like we originally thought.[68]

For instance, the immune cells that are present at the implantation site were assumed to be a response to the presence of a "foreign" fetus. Research has indicated that this may not actually be the case—instead, it may be an indication that the mother's immune system is working extra hard to protect the baby from external harm.[69] The unique immunological protection provided by the placenta itself is also being uncovered, leading to the realization that the fetus is actively being kept more safe than we thought.

Two particular areas of the body that undergo inflammatory changes during pregnancy may be responsible for the subsequent onset of autoimmune disorders. The thyroid becomes more active during pregnancy and must supply the fetus for the first couple of months. The inflammation caused by this event may be a trigger involved in the frequent onset of hypothyroidism during or after pregnancy. Secondly, an aptly named hormone called *relaxin* begins to be released into the body, partly to prevent the uterus from beginning contractions too early, but also to allow the joints to become more pliable—preparing the way for an easier childbirth. The inflammation created as these joints return to their normal state may be a trigger for the connective tissue disorders such as rheumatoid arthritis often seen after pregnancy.

Seasonal Changes

There are many people who report a seasonal aspect to the nature of their disease. In the Lujan et. al study I mentioned earlier, where they injected aluminum into the sheep in an attempt to track the metal's movement, the symptoms the sheep experienced were markedly worse during the winter. Besides the risk of upsetting aluminum-containing granulomas, how might wintertime affect the severity of man-made disease?

Decreased sunlight may play a part. Sunlight helps your body produce vitamin D, a component of the immune system, and diseases like ALS and SAD (seasonal affective disorder) seem to be more prominent as you move further north or south from the equator, where direct exposure is reduced. Similarly, the shorter daylight hours of winter may manipulate your production of vitamin D. The interaction between vitamin D and your immune system is fairly complex and is discussed more thoroughly in the chapter "The Problem with Vitamin D."

Viral and bacterial infections also tend to peak in winter, possibly due to more people being indoors and encouraging their spread. The increased immunological challenge presented by wintertime may tilt the balance in favor of the intracellular bacteria your body fights on a day to day basis.

Another possibility is linked to the pineal gland, a part of your brain that creates melatonin in response to light and dark cycles during the day. Melatonin is a hormone that helps your body ready itself for sleep, and the pineal gland has been shown to accumulate more than twice the aluminum than other brain tissues.[70] Perhaps the disruption to sleep patterns that come with shortened daylight hours—not to mention the antiquated daylight savings time shift—play a larger role in your immune system health than we realize.

Whatever the reason, the simple fact these diseases can come and go from various environmental factors should convince anyone they are not genetic inevitabilities, but an active attempt by your body to rid itself of an infection.

WHAT'S IN A NAME?

I remember first learning about clouds when I was in the 4th grade. There were three types of clouds: Stratus, Cumulus and Nimbus. We glued different cotton ball shapes onto blue construction paper to illustrate them. When I got a little older, I saw other shapes. There weren't just three cotton balls anymore, but many variations of each. In 9th grade, we learned there weren't just three shapes, but were in fact many more. New types of clouds hadn't been invented during this time, but because we had gotten older, our capability for specificity had increased. If you were to study meteorology in college, you may learn the names for hundreds of different cloud formations. This knowledge will allow you to make better informed decisions about what the weather is likely to do in the future.

The way in which we name and label modern illness has followed a similar pattern over the last one hundred years. In the past, a disease was most often caused by a virus or bacteria. This pathogen created a distinct set of symptoms that allowed anyone to easily identify the cause of sickness. Red blotchy skin rash—measles. Itch, blister-like rash

—chickenpox. A diagnosis was easy.

With traditional disease, there was an onset of illness associated with the initial infection. As your body fought off the infection, it would generate symptoms. Within a few days, your body would usually create enough antibodies to kill off the invader—at which point your symptoms would go away, possibly never to bother you again. Everyone, especially physicians trained in the classical methods, tend to think of modern disease within this framework—onset, symptoms, healing, health. With modern disease, this sequence of events is disrupted. Parts of your body may be kept in a constant state of inflammation and your immune system is unable to gain the upper hand. Any number of events may bring the inflammation under control, only for them to come back in another part of your body.

When you have been suffering from serious illness, it can feel like a huge relief to be given a diagnosis for the constellation of symptoms you've been experiencing. It can give you assurance that you are not going to die by learning about other people who are thriving and have found ways to cope with the same illness. It's also comforting just to know that you are not alone—that there are other people out there with similar symptoms as yourself.

As you become more familiar with your diagnosis, you will start to find gaps in the description. You will see a common symptom or two that you don't have. And then, you'll realize that a serious problem you developed alongside your initial diagnosis doesn't appear to affect anyone else. You may scan stories and videos looking for someone just like you but are unable to find them. Maybe your diagnosis was wrong, you'll think to yourself. Maybe there's a different disease out there that properly represents who you are, and for that diagnosis maybe there will be more effective treatment. And to complicate matters, during the year or two that you've struggled for a correct diagnosis, the symptoms have changed. What felt like pins and needles are now deep muscle aches. What felt like general fatigue now seems more like brain fog.

Man-made diseases can be some of the hardest illnesses to deal with psychologically. Doctors will often have a difficult time giving you a diagnosis because of the overlap in symptoms you're likely to experience. A change in your symptoms from month to month can make it nearly impossible. Naming and labeling these modern disorders is like sitting under a sky full of clouds and trying to come up with a single name for all of them—if you take too long, the formation will have changed and you will need to start all over.

From hundreds of years of medical history, it's been ingrained in our heads that an illness is due to a specific cause. It used to be a virus or bacteria that was causing the problem. For modern disease, we're told we don't know what the cause is and we can't even clearly define the symptoms—it's a real conundrum we've created.

This is a common path many suffer through as they try to come to terms with their suffering—What is my illness called? What are the treatment options? If you are just going through this journey now, there is bad news and good news within the answer to those statements. The bad news is—modern medicine unfortunately has very few ideas about healing most of these illnesses. They have plenty of medicine to help deal with the symptoms, but because they don't understand the cause, they cannot address the underlying conditions.

Emotionally, a diagnosis can feel like everything. Connecting with other people like yourself and being able to gain a strong support network when friends and family may have failed you is absolutely essential—a diagnosis can help you find those people. But the good news is—the diagnosis may not matter. The cause of modern disease may be the same one or two things. If this is true, it will mean that whatever the diagnoses are, they can be healed the same way.

The next part of the book will go through many of the man-made diseases and attempt to explain what might be causing them. For clarity, I have listed them by their common names, but I want to reiterate that I think these labels are misleading. They may give you the indication that you have a particular disease with particular symptoms and that it is unlikely to change. With most, the symptoms will shift from place to place as the infections that are taking in place in their body rise and fall. For this reason, many are likely to cycle through various components of many of the illnesses listed.

I will start explaining the disorders by first going through the ones I attribute to acute neurological damage – these are mostly issues caused by problems with the cranial nerves. Then I'll go through a few other diseases, disorders and syndromes, many of which would be placed in the category of autoimmune. I recommend you avoid using the next section as a reference initially. Try to read through it completely as most chapters mention new concepts that might not be covered elsewhere.

DISEASES OF METAL

The eye sees only what the mind is prepared to comprehend.

— Robertson Davies

    This section goes through many disorders which may be caused by acute metal toxicity alone—no microbes required. You will notice these are mostly neurological issues. While chronic infections can play a part in neurological disease, the next few chapters will be spent explaining how neurotoxins like aluminum may cause these illnesses.

CROOKED SMILES

"It has been presumed, that the act of smiling is peculiar to the human countenance, and that in no other creature can there arise that state of enjoyment which produces this distinguishing character of the human face, the affection of benevolence, or the enjoyment of the ridiculous. But every one must have observed how near the approach is to this expression in a dog, when he fawns on his master, and leaps and twists his body and wags his tail, while at the same time he turns out the edge of the lips as like a laugh as his organs can express."[71]

— *Charles Bell, The Nervous System of the Human Body*

When you begin to spot crooked smiles, one thing you will undoubtedly notice, especially in babies, is the entire side of their face looks different—it's not just the mouth. When you smile, the act of pulling the side of your mouth upwards and outwards makes your cheeks puff out. You can see this on your own face even without a mirror—when you smile you may notice your cheeks come in and out of view of the bottom of your eye.

Because of these cheek movements, your eyes close slightly—not from the eyelid moving downward, but from the bottom of your eye moving upward. Illustrators and animators will instinctively draw "happy eyes" in this shape, where the bottom of the eye lid curves up. Photographers call this "squinching", which is different than "squinting." Squinting is bringing both eyelids together—it can signify anger or suspicion.[i] The difference between a dull portrait and a vibrant one can often be attributed to learning how to squinch your eyes— bringing up the bottom of your eye without having to smile to do it.

When anyone smiles, especially a baby who typically has chubby cheeks, you should see their eyes close from the bottom upwards. If you see a picture of them smiling and notice that one eye looks bigger than the other, this might be because the cheek on that side is not pulling up properly. I often hear parents remark at seeing an asymmetrical picture of their child—at how one side of their baby's face looks like it's swollen shut.

"Like they got stung by a bee," a mother said to me.

The side of their face with the "bee sting" is actually how they're supposed to look—they are showing happiness on that side of their face. It's the opposite side that's not working. If you cover the open-eyed side of the picture, you can see they are just showing the typical face of a very happy baby. When only one side is doing it, it looks inherently wrong—like they got stung by a bee.

Once I began to recognize the mechanical flaw, it became obvious when babies were not able to smile on one side. It wasn't just the corner of their mouth curving up and backwards towards their ear, and it

---

i. Squinting can also be an attempt to correct one's vision, as George Constanza would insist on in Seinfeld episode 67, "The Glasses." There is some evidence squinting can actually correct vision to a degree as the action bends the lens of the eye and allows for better focus.

wasn't just the fact that one of their eyes was squinching while the other stayed wide open. It was the absence of what is called a nasal labial fold —the crease that runs from the bottom corner of your nose down past the side of your mouth.

A pronounced nasal labial fold is easily visible in older people, presumably the badge of a lifetime of happiness. On babies, this fold is usually absent until they smile. If the fold is absent on one side, *and* you can account for differences in lighting and shadow, it may indicate that one side of their face is not working like it should. When they smile, if you spot the absence of the nasal labial fold on one side and their eye on that same side appears to be more rounded, you may assume they have some facial palsy.

A quick note about smirking—that sly, cheeky half-smile that so many attribute our Hollywood crooked faces to. It can be difficult to differentiate a smirk from a truly crooked smile caused by facial palsy, but there is one technique I sometimes use.

A crooked smile happens because one side of the face is working poorly. It doesn't mean there is complete paralysis, but enough general muscle weakness that it makes smiling straight difficult. Natalie Dormer has mentioned in interviews that if she concentrates, she can smile straight. But because of weakness on the left side of her face, she naturally smiles up on the right, down on the left. What people assume is her "smirking" is so noticeable they get annoyed with it, so she addressed it in comments and tried to explain to people she isn't making that face on purpose. It's her natural smile. With a lot of work, she can smile more symmetrically. Daniel Radcliffe is the same way. His natural smile features muscle weakness on the right side (uncommon), rather than the left. He evidently has put a lot of effort into learning to smile symmetrically and you can almost see the strain in his face in pictures of him smiling straight.

This is why you will see many people sometimes smile crooked, and other times straight. It may not be permanent or always visible, but with effort, some people with facial palsy can smile straight. When they are tired, or perhaps not concentrating on their smile, it will sometimes be off to the side.

A true smirk might require both sides of the face to be working. If you are smirking towards the right side of your face (most common), the left side of your mouth—the top and bottom left lips—will pull over along with the right. The natural effect of this motion is your mouth will close and the bottom left of your nose will swing over towards the right. If I see a sideways smile with an open mouth and the nose appears to have not moved much, it will point towards facial palsy. If the mouth is closed, and the nose appears to have pulled over, I might assume smirk.

It is foolish to suppose there is a binary decision tree that would allow someone to determine what is a smirk and what is true facial palsy from a photograph, but these details may be useful to someone who is going back through their childhood photographs to try and determine when they developed a crooked smile. With video, the effects I have described become more pronounced and determination of whether it is a smirk or a truly crooked smile becomes easier.

CROOKED EYES

Parents will often notice their child's eyes becoming misaligned long before they notice anything else in their face. A crooked smile might warm some parents hearts, but when eyes begin pointing in different directions, parents instinctively think there might be a problem. I searched the message boards to find out what parents were making of their children's misaligned eyes and messages like the following were common:

> *"Posting here as I feel a bit overwhelmed and I just want to burst into tears at the moment. My dd (dear daughter) turned 18 months and noticed since she was 9 months old one of her eyes turns outwards. I immediately flagged to the pediatrician who said no concerns and we need to wait it out. I was not convinced and I went to an ophthalmologist who checked my baby at that age and said nothing to worry … At some point the wandering eye disappeared and reappeared on both eyes some three months ago. I again took her to ophthalmologist who said it's too early to say anything and that we need to come back*

when she's 24 months old or older. He did only visual examination. I wasn't convinced and took to another doctor for second opinion. The latter told the same that if she had problems we will be able to detect it only once she's a bit older. He also added that in any case if it's a problem with eye vision it will be corrected with glasses but once she's a bit older and that now she won't allow me to put glasses on her … I just have a feeling that doctors are not taking my concerns seriously!!!! I am very concerned that if we continue 'let's wait and see' practice we might lose the opportunity to correct anything from a young age … I am turning to you ladies to see if anyone has been in similar situation? Thanks a lot and I really appreciate getting some opinions here. I am a first time mom and I feel so worried!!"

The despair this mom was feeling because her concerns were being ignored is unfortunately all too common. Here maternal instincts were screaming to her that something was wrong, but they weren't taken seriously. Unsatisfied with the first doctor response, she took her daughter to a specialist. The specialist appeared to think it was nothing and so she went to a third doctor, hoping for answers. The fact that her daughter's eye appeared to correct itself, then re-appeared is a definite cause for concern that should have triggered an alert in any physician. I am not aware of muscle weakness that comes and goes—and then comes back again. Something was causing her daughter's eye to deviate, and the three doctors she went to appeared uninterested in finding out why.

It's interesting that exotropic strabismus—where an eye deviates outwards—is not as noticeable. For some reason, when an eye points inward—called esotropic strabismus—it is an effect that is instantly recognizable. We even have a term, a derogatory term actually, "cross-eyed" that every kid learns as they grow up for this type of strabismus.

Because the inward and outward motions of your eyes are

controlled by separate muscles, it would seem that you could purposefully cross them outwards just as well as inwards. Apparently, because your eyes have to cross when you look at an object up close and never deviate outwards (at the same time) beyond simply straight ahead, our brain hasn't developed the ability to deviate both eyes outward. I have heard of a few people with a special talent that can pull this feat off, but I personally have never seen anyone be able to do it.

Part of the reason doctors are frequently unconcerned with such an issue is because it *will* often resolve itself. With today's modern healthcare practices emphasizing quantity over quality, pediatricians have limited time with their patients anyway and are keen to triage any patient that comes in quickly. In their years of experience, they have probably seen this problem come and go many times and realize that it often does go away. The fact that they don't know why it appears *or* disappears is no comfort to anyone, and as we will learn later on, unexplained phenomena like this should make any physician question why it's happening—regardless as to whether it seems to be a trivial issue or not. The unknown can be a dangerous thing.

RIGHT SIDE HIGH. LEFT SIDE LOW.

After looking at thousands of crooked faces, I was still noticing that most people displayed facial palsy on their left side. I had even found scientific research that seemed to confirm it, but was unable to come up with any plausible reason why it was happening. As I began to understand the nature of aluminum transport within the body, a completely plausible answer appeared out of nowhere. The reason for the prevalence of left-side paralysis became clear and convinced me I was on the right path with some of my other theories.

From the research I had read, I knew that aluminum was seen as an invader, and white blood cells, the body's frontline defense mechanism, attacked them as they would any other pathogen. Unlike a naturally occurring virus or bacteria, aluminum could not be destroyed. So the white blood cells would circulate in the blood, carrying the aluminum along with them until they came to rest, typically within muscle tissue or occasionally granulomas.

There are actually two circulatory systems in the body—the cardiovascular, which circulates blood, and the lymphatic system, an integral part of the immune system. The lymphatic system is missing something very important that the cardiovascular has—a pump. The heart is a powerful organ that circulates blood throughout the body—60,000 miles of arteries, veins and capillaries. The lymphatic system has no such organ to pump it's fluid around the body and depends on movement for circulation. Much like a self-winding clock, as long as your body has motion, your lymphatic system will circulate properly, helping your immune system to function at its best. This is why people who are sick and laid up in bed would benefit from some sort of daily activity. If they can move their arms, kick their legs or walk in place, they should—this tiny bit of exercise will keep their lymphatic system flowing and improve the function of their immune system.

Knowing that aluminum can circulate through the body in both the cardiovascular and lymphatic systems, you might be inclined to take a look at a diagram of the flow of these networks. In the cardiovascular system, you will find a vast array of arteries that carry blood away from the heart, splitting and forking into smaller and smaller vessels until they become capillaries, where the oxygen carried by the blood is actually delivered to tissue through the body. After the capillaries, the vessels become veins that return oxygen-depleted blood back to the heart.

A typical diagram of the cardiovascular system, besides the peculiar layout of the internal organs, is mainly symmetrical as it extends into the extremities and brain. The lymph system is very different. For reasons that are not known, the human lymphatic system is decidedly asymmetrical. Extremely crooked, one might say.

The two sections of the lymphatic system are named by the ducts that drain lymph back into the cardiovascular system. One side drains through what is called the *lymphatic duct* and it covers the upper right torso and arm. The other side, referred to by the *thoracic duct* through which it drains, covers the rest of the body—the left upper torso, the left arm, the entire abdomen and both legs. This unusual layout creates a lot of lymphatic tissue that might seem to drain into the left side of your heart. Without explaining what might be going on, I had found at least something significant—an asymmetrical system within the body which we know is capable of transporting white blood cells—white blood cells containing aluminum and possibly other toxins.

Another clue emerged as I researched the actual administration of vaccines. I asked some nurses anonymously online plus a few I knew personally if they had been taught to administer shots in a particular arm—left or right. One replied that they gave the shot in the dominant arm.

She said, "The more you use the muscle, the faster the medication will be distributed which will make it less painful. Eventually, it all gets absorbed no matter which arm is used."

Her answer would later haunt me, as I came to understand the mechanism by which the "medication" as she called it was *not* absorbed.[72] Most of the other answers I received indicated a left arm preference.

"Vaccines can cause localized muscle pain," another nurse told me, "and it just makes sense not to cause unnecessary pain in an arm that a person needs to use frequently. If a person is left handed, they need to be sure to let the health care professional know prior to injection so they will inject the right arm."

It was starting to make sense why the left side might get more of the toxins from vaccines injected, but what about babies? They were too young to show a left or right-side dominance. Were they still injected in their left arm anyway?

"Do you imagine infants & toddlers," I asked, "who may not have a hand preference yet, would receive shots in their left more often simply out of habit?"

One of the nurses responded with an answer that made it all too clear why so many were developing left side paralysis. "Vaccines are usually given in the thigh muscle for infants as the arm does not have sufficient muscle mass yet."

In our asymmetrical lymphatic system, most of the body is dedicated to the "left" side. More importantly, both legs, the injection sites for infants, were channeled into this side. I went online and found illustrations of how to simultaneously administer multiple vaccines at once to a baby. The subcutaneous injection could be given in the arm, but the four intra-muscular injections would all be given in their legs—all areas that would funnel into the left side of the lymphatic system. And to further intrigue me, I realized the subcutaneous shot—the inactivated polio vaccine—didn't contain any metal, but all four of the intra-muscular shots—the pneumococcal, Hepatitis B, Hib and DTaP shots—all contain aluminum.[73]

It wouldn't matter which arm received the polio shot. The other four injections, the ones administered in an infant's legs—all had aluminum. And all of the aluminum would funnel into the left side of the lymphatic system.

If you research the lymphatic system, you will easily find asymmetric diagrams of their flow. But you may also notice something else—most all of them will stop at the neck. Some will show the lymphatic system extend above the neck and around the sides of the head, but curiously, never the brain itself. This was because the lymphatic system is believed to not extend into the brain—a notion which presented a problem. If there *was* some association between the left-side prevalence of facial asymmetry and the similarly asymmetrical lymphatic system, how could that be if the lymphatic system never actually reached the brain? In 2015 and 2016, researchers from the University of Virginia School of Medicine and the National Institutes of Health would make two incredible discoveries that would forever change how we thought about the brain and the lymphatic system.

LYMPH IN THE BRAIN

In 2003, five authors reviewed a massive collection of 867 anatomical models in the Josephinum Wax Model Museum in Vienna, Austria. The collection includes haunting partial and full body sculptures of humans, their organs, their diseases and death. The purpose of the article was to critique four of the models which stood out "for their obvious anatomical misconceptions."

One of the models in question was done by Paolo Mascagni, an Italian physician born just twenty years before Charles Bell. Like Bell, he was fascinated by anatomy and had spent considerable effort creating wax models of the human body, even going so far as to develop a technique of injecting mercury to aid in visualizing the lymph vessels.[74] Mascagni was capable of producing models of incredible fidelity and accuracy, so it was with great aplomb the authors felt the need to critique one of his sculptures—Showcase 251/1: Inferior aspect of the brain with the arteries, lymph vessels, and the origin of nerves.

The authors remarked, "Mascagni was probably so impressed with the lymphatic system that he saw lymph vessels even where they did not exist—the human brain."[75]

The caption to their photo of Mascagni's brain model highlighted his error in case they weren't clear: "Note lymph vessels on the brain surface."[76]

Mascagni's work was warmly received by the scientific community initially, but sometime after his anatomical models were made, it was decided that the brain did not actually have a lymphatic system. Although it was an organ like the liver or spleen, scientists could not readily see a lymphatic system in the brain and therefore determined it did not exist. The brain seemingly thrived despite occupying an immunological vacuum, devoid of the dense network of vessels responsible for delivering and carrying away the detritus of neurological healing.

Despite the hundreds of thousands of additional cadavers studied, charts drawn, and anatomical models created since Mascagni's sculpture in the late 1700s, no one spotted any sign of lymphatic tissue in the brain. Every chart available on the planet showed the lymphatic system stopping somewhere in the upper neck. It was as if Mascagni had seen and mapped a super human who had once walked the planet but would never again exist. This would all change in 2015.

"I thought the body was mapped." Jonathan Kipnis, a professor and director of the University of Virginia's Center for Brain Immunology and Glia, was astounded as the results of their latest research became apparent.

Kipnis and a postdoctoral fellow on his team figured out a way to delicately remove the meninges, the membrane which covers the brain, from a mouse. They were then able to mount the membrane onto a slide and perform some tests for lymphatic tissue. They may have not been inspired so much by Mascagni's 200-year old work, but rather a simple hunch that if the other organs in the body employed lymphatic vessels for their health, why wouldn't the brain?

They were astonished by what they saw. "They'll have to rewrite the textbooks," remarked one of their colleagues who first saw the results.[77] It was clear—the meninges had a complex network of lymphatic vessels that spidered across the membrane that had been carefully laid onto the slide.

Around the same time, a team from the NIH Neurological Disorders and Strokes group, led by neuroradiologist Daniel Reich, had developed a method to detect minute lymphatic vessels with MRI.[78] This new technique would allow them to see inside the brain—a human brain, and a living one at that—to create a much more complete picture of the lymphatic network within—assuming it existed.

Like the group from Virginia, they were also amazed at the matrix of lymphatic tissue that appeared on their computer screens, a gossamer tangle of green that must have been intricately woven through every human brain since the beginning of time, though no one had even been able to see it. Mascagni's sculpture—well over two-hundred years old—had been right all along.

The left side prevalence of cranial nerve damage, particularly facial palsy, had a plausible reason, as far as I was concerned. The lymphatic system was divided into two separate parts. One side, the *lymphatic duct* side might capture and circulate injected toxins from the right arm. The other half, the *thoracic duct* side, would capture and circulate injected toxins from everywhere else—the left arm and both legs. Most vaccines are administered in children's legs, where there is more muscle tissue. If metal was being transported into the brain via the lymphatic system, we should expect to see left side damage more than the right.

And that's exactly what I had seen. Up on the right. Down on the left. Almost every time.

ADHD

For years, people have told parents of children with ADHD that they just need to get outside and play more—that sitting still in chairs for hours at school is not natural for children to have to do—especially for boys. A parent might respond, "No, this is different. Something's not right with them—it's not boredom from sitting still for too long—it's an uncontrollable energy that goes beyond fidgeting or restlessness."

If you're an adult who has been diagnosed with ADHD, you may have found it easier to cope with these issues as you have matured. Depending on the severity of your disorder, you may have learned how to mask your symptoms so completely that no one would even know you have it. Other adults, for whom their symptoms are severe, can struggle with depression, anxiety and drug abuse. Regardless, for the estimated 7% of children[79] who are just learning how to control their emotions and the limits of socially acceptable behavior, ADHD can be very difficult. The emotional toll these challenges can put on children and their families is often trivialized in light of the suffering of "real" disorders such as autism.

If you have sensed that something is not right with your child's behavior and had others dismiss your anxiety as over-concern, you are not alone. Parents the world over have experienced the behaviors of their hyperactive kids, realized that something wasn't right, spoken up about it to a trusted friend or physician, only to have their concerns brushed aside.

Some children have a very clear issue with paying attention, speaking out inappropriately, fidgeting, wiggling, and many other behaviors that make their lives extremely challenging. Many of these kids may experience social issues due to not being able to make friends at school, not being asked to birthday parties, or tremendous anxiety from realizing that something is "different" about them.

When you experience a child exhibiting these symptoms, it can be as obvious a diagnosis as someone who stutters. I believe there is a physiological issue causing these behaviors—it's not boredom or not enough stimulation, but something clearly misfiring in the brain. I think ADHD is caused by damage from either chronic inflammation or metal toxicity in a specific part of the brain called the *locus coeruleus*.

The locos coeruleus is a small area inside the brain stem that is responsible for responding to stress or panic. It initiates the production of *norepinephrine*, a substance that works to prepare your body for fight or flight by increasing alertness and improving your ability to store and retrieve memory. This sequence of events is an aggressive chemical response to a perceived threat. When the locus coeruleus is damaged, it may be hypersensitive and interpret trivial environmental events as cues for possible danger. It may also emit constant signals for norepinephrine production. This hormone may be necessary during a true threat, but a constant stream of norepinephrine in the body can cause many of the same symptoms we associate with ADHD.[80] It's also why children with ADHD frequently have horrible gut issues—all energy is being diverted away from digestion and immune response towards preparing their body for battle.

Is the problem due to chronic inflammation, or just metal toxicity? As with most of the disorders mentioned in the book, we can assume that metals are involved either way. Studies have shown increased levels of metal, including aluminum, in the hair of children diagnosed with hyperactivity.[81] In an infant's head, the locus coeruleus is less than half an inch away from many of the other cranial nerve nuclei that may be damaged by aluminum. In a child with other signs of cranial nerve damage, it would not be much of a stretch to presume that their locus coeruleus also has lesions.

For this reason, I believe that many children who exhibit ADHD behaviors have some damage from acute metal toxicity. If you have noticed your child's symptoms improve during a fever, this may lead you to believe their condition is due to inflammation. While I cannot say what is causing your child's condition, the positive effects of fever may have little to do with inflammation abatement and more to do with a temporary respite from norepinephrine overdosing.[i]

Teachers and school administrators should be glad to know ADHD has nothing to do with not enough smart boards or a stale classroom experience. Parents should be ecstatic to know that the behaviors their children are exhibiting may be lessened, if not completely cleared, with a lot of patience and the metal chelation therapies mentioned in the healing and recovery chapter of this book.

---

i. See the next chapter "Why Fevers Improve Autism/ADHD Symptoms." for more information on this phenomenon.

FEVERS IMPROVE AUTISM/ADHD?

Many parents of children with autism or ADHD have noticed a strange phenomenon—their children's behaviors will improve dramatically with a fever. The reason I believe this effect is happening should give parents a tremendous amount of hope their children can improve—permanently.

With an especially challenging child, sick days can be difficult. For a stressed out mother with younger children to take care of, the break a few hours of school provides her can mean everything. When one of their children gets sick, the parent may dread having to nurse and soothe them while handling their behavioral issues at the same time. I've heard many stories like this:

> *"(Sam) was grumpy—more than normal and didn't want to wake up. He was running a fever and I thought, 'Not today. Please not today.' He had an epic meltdown the night before and I was exhausted. I had so much to get done and was going to try and sneak a nap in if I could and now he was going to have to*

stay home from school. I was so pissed. But then something weird happened. He ate his breakfast. There was no battle. He sat down, and ate it, as if he'd just taken a Xanax or something. He was so chill. I sat down with him on the couch and asked him if he felt okay. He said his head hurt and he was sleepy. I turned on a movie and we watched it for two hours! We talked about the movie while we were watching it. He asked me questions! He never asks me questions. I was going to give him some Tylenol but couldn't believe how different he was. That was probably the best day we've had since he was diagnosed."

As the fever abated, Sam's symptoms returned and his difficult behaviors began again. This sequence of events happens so frequently that scientists have studied its effects in an attempt to unlock the mysteries of autism and ADHD. If you peer through the literature on this subject, you may find the possible explanations to be obtuse:

"We hypothesize that febrigenesis and the behavioral-state changes associated with fever in autism depend upon selective normalization of key components of a functionally impaired locus coeruleus-noradrenergic (LC-NA) system. We posit that autistic behaviors result from developmental dysregulation of LC-NA system specification and neural network deployment and modulation linked to the core behavioral features of autism. Fever transiently restores the modulatory functions of the LC-NA system and ameliorates autistic behaviors."[82]

The locus coeruleus is partly responsible for managing your response to stress by increasing the production of norepinephrine, but it has another important job—it manages your body's response to fever. Like many functions in the brain, it is poorly understood. However, it's clear that the locus coeruleus plays an important role in modulating your body during a fever.

I believe many of the behavioral issues associated with ASD and ADHD are due to children being locked in a panicked, high-anxiety state of fight or flight due to inappropriate releases of cortisol or norepinephrine. When someone is in this state, most of their body's energy is directed away from their gut and immune system. This is why so many of these children have bowel issues—their body is using as little energy as possible for digestion in an attempt to reserve energy to protect themselves. Their immune system may also suffer, giving rise to frequent ear infections and other illnesses.

Two things happen during a fever that can help a child with autism or ADHD feel better. First off, the body senses that the immune system is going to need help and begins to divert resources away from the fight or flight state. Secondly, the majority of norepinephrine the body is making is directed by the locus coeruleus into producing the effects of a fever—by raising the body temperature.[83] The amount of energy it takes to raise the core temperature of the body by several degrees is tremendous and has the effect of cutting off the over-production of norepinephrine the child experiences every day.

Within hours, they experience the effects of having normal norepinephrine levels in their body. Calm. Attentive. Capable of sitting still. No outbursts. As if they are a different child. Unfortunately, within hours of the fever leaving their body, the effects of too much norepinephrine surface again.

This hypothetical explanation should give you a tremendous amount of hope that your child's symptoms can be lessened. If your child has ADHD or is on the autism spectrum and you have experienced this effect, you can see what a massive difference modulating this one factor makes. They may have other issues that will have their own set of challenges, but getting your children's locus coeruleus clear of metal should be a priority for anyone who has seen this effect in their children.

SPEECH DISORDERS

No. LVII

In consequence of your important discoveries relative to the nerves, I am particularly desirous to have your opinion on the following case. From the first of her complaining to the present moment, she has been free from headache and from pain, numbness, or debility of the limbs. The vision and hearing are natural; the appetite good; the bowels regular, and the sleep natural. Some few months ago she had some difficulty in using the tongue, and in expressing particular words. This difficulty has gradually increased, and now she cannot protrude the tongue, or even move it. She has lost her speech altogether… occasionally she is distressed with a sense of suffocation, in attempting to swallow food, which she is now obliged to do with great care. She cannot hack up any thing from the throat, nor draw any thing from the posterior nares by a back draught.[i]

* * *

---

i. *The modern term for this would be "hocking up a lugey."*

An issue that can arise from problems with cranial nerves is a speech disorder. There are several different ways in which cranial nerve damage might affect someone's speech and I want to go through all of them because I could see how speech therapists might miss these diagnoses.

If your child begins to demonstrate trouble talking, therapists will work with you to figure out what's wrong with them. One of the diagnoses they may give is called *apraxia of speech*. Apraxia refers to difficulty planning motor tasks. It can affect other things, like movement or gesturing, but in kids, it's often seen manifested as a speech disorder. It is thought that apraxia is caused by a lesion in the *posterior parietal cortex* of the brain. I only mention this location because I believe speech disorders often originate from somewhere else —the brain stem and the cranial nerves that emanate from there. Lesions on any number of cranial nerves can prevent proper speech.

I want to demonstrate all of the different cranial nerves that need to be functioning correctly in order for you to say a simple word: "Gandalf."[ii] For most of us, it takes no thought at all to form this word. Say it out loud: "Gandalf."

The word starts with the inhalation of air. You will need air pressure to produce the sounds used in this word, so before you can even begin to say this word, you must fill your lungs with a bit of air. Before the air comes out, two things happen. The back of your tongue has to lift up into the roof of your mouth so that it can temporarily stop the flow of air from the lungs. This requires the action of a few cranial nerves—the 12th to move your tongue up into the roof of your mouth, the 10th (and possibly the 9th) to help close the airway completely.

Your diaphragm begins to expel air against this seal but at the same time, a branch of the 10th vagus nerve causes your vocal chords to

---

ii. Gandalf the Grey is a wizard from J.R.R. Tolkien's "The Hobbit" and The Lord of the Rings series of books. Also a cat.

tighten and vibrate—this causes an actual sound to form. At this point, before your tongue releases the build-up of air behind it, the sound is just a shapeless tone within our body. Your 12th and 10th cranial nerves suddenly release the tongue from the roof of the mouth, creating the hiss of air as it escapes past the seal. The tone created by your vocal chords also comes out along with it and you've just made a "G" sound.

If you were making this sound in slow motion as you read along, you will probably have actually made a "guh" sound as in the word "gun." We actually need to make a "gan" sound as in "gander", and to do that, we need to change the shape of our mouth completely. This requires not only more coordination from the 12th cranial nerve and portions of the 10th, but also the 7th—the facial cranial nerve. The 7th controls the muscles that stretch out your cheeks to change the shape inside your mouth. We also need to open our mouth, requiring use of the 5th cranial nerve.

The "n" is made by stopping the flow of air again, this time with the front of the tongue instead of the back (5th to close the jaw, 7th to change the shape of the mouth, 10th to vibrate the vocal chords, and 12th to shape the tongue).

I will stop there, because we've required the use of 5, possibly 6 out of the 12 cranial nerves just to say half of a word. The "d" has its own requirements, as does the "al" vowel-consonant combination and the "f" at the end.

If your child has issues with their 9th cranial nerve, you may notice a nasal quality to their speech as they have trouble preventing air from exiting through their nose while they talk. If they have issues with their 10th cranial nerve, you may notice weakness and tremors in their voice as their vocal chords have trouble forming or holding the correct shapes. If they have issues with their 12th cranial nerve, their tongue control may be poor and a number of different sounds could be difficult for them to make.

The "y" sound, as in "yellow," is complex and requires both sides of the tongue to curl upwards, leaving a pathway for air to escape down the middle. If they have trouble making a "y" sound and prefer to use the tip their tongue instead by saying "lellow", this may indicate 12th cranial nerve palsy.

If your child consistently substitutes an incorrect sound, like saying "tree" instead of "three", this may indicate a 12th cranial nerve palsy rather than apraxia. "Th" is a difficult sound to make if your tongue muscles are not working perfectly. Add another consonant—the "r" at the end—and "three" becomes a very difficult word to pronounce without full control of both your tongue and cheek muscles. Inconsistent substitutions are more indicative of problems outside the cranial nerves.

As you deconstruct the mechanics of speech, you will realize that you talk with your face and neck muscles as much as you do your tongue—this is why people with hearing disabilities can learn to "read lips." They're not actually reading lips, of course, they're reading faces—from the opening and closing of the jaw, the shape of the cheeks and lips, the movement of the tongue inside, all the way up to the eyebrows and head tilt.

Learning to speak requires their hearing to work properly, something which can be negatively affected by another cranial nerve palsy[iii]. Speech therapists may diagnose your child with apraxia and suggest something is wrong with the posterior parietal cortex, but a careful check of their cranial nerve function may reveal a different problem.

It is beyond the scope of this book to diagnose your child's speech impairment but if you notice a specific problem, you might be able to

---

iii. This phenomenon is covered in the Hearing Disorders chapter isolate it to a particular cranial nerve based on some of what I've shown. If you are reading this and are concerned your child may develop a speech disorder, make sure you look at the guide at the back of this book to learn how to easily watch for signs of metal toxicity in your child's cranial nerve functions.

The cranial nerves that give your child the ability to speak can be damaged by metals like aluminum. If you believe your child may have developed cranial nerve palsies, take a look through the last few chapters of this book for ideas on healing and recovery.

There is another type of speech problem which falls under the *dyspraxia* label—I mention this in the Hearing & Motion Disorders chapter.

VISION DISORDERS

One of the most common vision disorders associated with cranial nerve damage is *diplopia*, or double vision. When the eyes become misaligned, due to weakness in the muscles that control movement, your brain's vision center cannot combine the two images properly and it appears as though you are seeing two of everything.

When your eyes cannot maintain alignment throughout their range of motion, this is called *strabismus*. Besides the crooked smile, this is one of the most easily recognized signs of cranial nerve damage.

Problems with the 2nd cranial nerve, the optic nerve, might surface as issues with brightness perception, color acuity and contrast. This may be difficult to diagnose in a non-verbal child, but adults with 2nd cranial nerve palsy have described their vision as dim, foggy and trouble with differentiating colors.

As I mention elsewhere, children with autism seem to have extremely advanced visual perception of motion, twice as good as a typical child.[84] Given what we have seen about how cranial nerve issues tend to increase sensitivity in sensory nerves, it is not hard to imagine how a 2nd cranial nerve palsy might be the culprit.

Why do some children look off to the side?

You may have noticed children sometimes appearing to look at things out of the corners of their eyes. Given the social deficits common amongst those on the spectrum, this might be attributed simply to impaired social behavior, especially as it pertains to eye contact.[i] However, there are two specific cranial nerve issues that may trigger this behavior.

If a child develops strabismus, the sudden misalignment will cause them to see double. This effect is less pronounced the further away from the center of their field of view the object is. So in order to cause their brain less confusion, they may purposefully hold their gaze in such a way as to minimize significant objects occupying the center of their field of view.

Problems with the 2nd cranial nerve can cause similar vision issues. Although blurriness in the center of the vision field is more commonly associated with *macular degeneration*, I propose that optic cranial nerve palsies can also trigger this phenomenon, causing anything in the center of the field of view to be blurry, even unrecognizable. If this happens, it would make sense why someone might look slightly askew from an object.

Why do some children hold objects so close to their face?

A common behavior amongst children on the autism spectrum is a fascination with the particular component of an toy—a fixation on a tiny part rather than the whole. Physicians aren't sure why this happens, and there are very few theories that attempt to explain it.

This strange phenomenon might be explained by cranial nerve

---

i. Another more disturbing cause for avoiding eye contact is proposed in the section on the Dorsal Vagal Complex.

palsies. The 2nd cranial nerve is a part of the *accommodation reflex*, a mechanism of sight that conveys information for adjusting focus. The *ciliary muscle* is a ring of muscle that helps control the shape of the lens of the eye. Without thinking about it, when an object is brought close to your face, the 2nd cranial nerve detects this change and sends information to the 5th cranial nerve—the *trigeminal* nerve normally associated with sensation on your face.

The 5th cranial nerve isn't just a sensory nerve but also conveys motion to a few things—one of which is the ciliary muscle. If an issue were to appear in either the 2nd or 5th cranial nerves, this might cause problems with control of the lens on the eye. In a phenomenon similar to the cranial nerve palsy and stapedius muscle dysfunction that causes hyperacusis, a lesion on the 2nd or 5th cranial nerve might cause the lens to become over-flexed in such a way someone develops extreme *myopia*, or nearsightedness.

If this were to happen, they might see things in focus only if they were held extremely close to their face. The tiny details on the surface of a Thomas the Tank toy would be crystal clear, as if they were viewing them through a microscope.

You will often see pictures of children with autism, completely self-absorbed on the floor playing with a single toy. If they are experiencing extreme myopia because of a cranial nerve lesion, simply getting their head near the toy may not be close enough to bring it into focus. As a result, you will see them turn their head sideways and lay it flat, in order to get their eyes directly next to what they are playing with.

Why do some children's eyes flick side to side?

I believe this phenomenon, often called *nystagmus*, to be a motion disorder and is covered in the motion disorder chapter.

HEARING & MOTION DISORDERS

Hearing Disorders (hyperacusis)

With cranial nerve damage, hearing disorders typically will cause increased sensitivity rather than the opposite. Hearing disorders are horrible because you cannot turn off sound. It goes through walls and windows—it's everywhere. You can get black out curtains for light, and remove offensive odors from your house, but it is difficult to turn off sound. It has driven people mad enough to kill themselves.

Hyperacusis is simply described as a hypersensitivity to sound. A more nuanced description would say it creates an inability to distinguish foreground from background noises. In a slightly noisy setting such as a school classroom, listening to someone talk can be challenging. In an extremely noisy environment such as a restaurant, tremendous cognitive energy is spent plucking out the person's voice sitting directly across from you from all of the other conversations going on.

If you have a hard time imagining what this is like, think back to those psychedelic 3-D stereogram posters from the 1990s. With thought and a purposeful crossing of the eyes, the outline of a previously hidden image might appear—only to disappear with the slightest lapse in concentration. Imagine having to think that hard just to listen to someone talk—you can imagine how people with hyperacusis may prefer a quiet conversation with someone at home, where the background sound might be more easily controlled.

There are at least three potential causes for hyperacusis. A common one involves problems with the 7th cranial nerve. Although this cranial nerve is responsible for movement of the face, it also plays a role in your hearing. The 7th cranial nerve controls the *stapedius*, the tiniest muscle in the body which stabilizes the *stape* (often referred to as the *stirrup bone* in elementary school science class)—the smallest bone in the body.

When functioning properly, these two work together to dampen vibrations on a membrane that leads into your inner ear, preventing loud noises from damaging your hearing. If the stapedius becomes paralyzed, it can no longer stabilize the tiny bone and everything will sound louder, leading to a diagnosis of hyperacusis.

Interestingly, the stapedius muscle engages the stapes whenever you speak, reducing the volume of your own voice by around 20 decibels. This may have something to do with why a child who suddenly developed cranial nerve palsy might speak less than before—the increase in the volume of their own voice might be alarming.

The 8th cranial nerve is responsible for hearing and motion of the inner ear. It is a sensory nerve, and like most sensory nerves, issues tend to show up as hypersensitivities. If there is a palsy on the 8th cranial nerve, it may show up as hyperacusis.

Finally, dysfunction in the thalamus area of the brain can also cause this hypersensitivity. If both ears have developed this hypersensitivity the thalamus might be a more likely cause than cranial nerve nuclei—particularly if other senses have become heightened. If only one ear is affected, as is the case for some Bell's palsy patients, it would point to a simpler cranial nerve palsy. If a child has both hyperacusis and any of the motion disorders listed below, it might point to an 8th cranial nerve palsy.

Motion Disorders (toe-walking, spinning, and nystagmus, clumsiness, dyspraxia)

In addition to hearing, the 8th cranial nerve is responsible for conveying balance and motion from the vestibular system to your brain. Problems with this cranial nerve can cause hypersensitivities that show up in a few seemingly unrelated ways.

Toe walking is a very common sight amongst children with autism, and people have always wondered why they do this. Theories have ranged from shortened leg muscles to sensory problems with the heels of their feet. I believe toe walking is a response to an 8th cranial nerve palsy manifested as hypersensitivity to vertical motion. If you've ever seen a cartoon of someone trying to sneak around, you will no doubt have noticed them walking on their toes. Walking this way creates less noise. Why? Because the heel-toe strikes of normal walking are much more dramatic.

Walking is falling forward and catching yourself over and over. When you walk on your toes, this falling effect is minimized and your weight distribution is more constant. The next time you see a cartoon of someone sneaking, watch their head. You will notice it stays even—it doesn't bob up and down like in a normal walk cycle. I believe children with a common type of hypersensitivity to motion walk on their toes because it reduces the disorientation caused by stepping normally. You could think of it like earmuffs for motion, rather than sound. Try walking both normally and on your toes on creaky floorboards—you will literally hear the difference.

* * *

Spinning in circles may be a compensational behavior caused by issues with the inner ear. Vertigo happens when the sensory inputs from your balance system don't align with what your eyes are seeing. It can create the intense feeling that you are moving or spinning. I believe children who like to spin in circles are actually trying to "unwind" the dizziness and vertigo they are experiencing. Their environment may feel like it is spinning around them from left to right, so they begin spinning left to right to offset the sensation. Because their eyes will betray this attempt at negating the spinning vertigo sensation, they will often look down on the ground to minimize the disconnect.

Nystagmus is a disorder of the eyes where they flick back and forth —most commonly side to side. This motion is involuntary, and although it looks disconcerting to someone watching the effect, people who experience this have grown accustomed to the motion and can read just fine.

What causes nystagmus? A component of your sense of balance is called the *vestibulo-ocular reflex.* This reflex coordinates the motion of your head with the nerves that control your eye positioning so that you can easily track objects in your field of view while your head is moving.

If you've ever seen someone hold an owl and move their body around, their remarkable vestibular-ocular reflex allows their head to stay perfectly locked on center. When there is a problem with this reflex, your brain may sense movement and make an adjustment to your eye positioning. Because there was actually no movement, once the eye has moved a tiny bit, the vision part of your brain realizes the error and moves the eye back to where it was. But the dysfunctional 8th cranial nerve is causing your brain to continually receive signals of motion so this adjustment and compensation sequence of moves continues over and over, causing your eyes to flick back and forth. An

8th cranial nerve palsy can also affect hearing—a fact that would explain why hearing problems are common in people with nystagmus.

Clumsiness is a symptom some children experience. Uncoordinated. Accident-prone. For parents who grew up active in sports, a child who has difficulty with simple eye-hand coordination tasks like catching a ball can seem baffling. Many will chalk up their children's awkwardness to genetic differences, but I believe there may be something physically wrong with some of these children—a condition which perhaps can be improved.

If you've noticed your child lose their sense of balance in a non-challenging situation such as walking or leaning against a door frame, this may point towards vertigo and cranial nerve problems. As mentioned above, issues with the 8th cranial nerve can give someone the sensation that they're moving even when they are not. Other parts of their body, such as their eyes, will indicate otherwise, and the brain tries to correct for this discrepancy. Sometimes, it doesn't work and they will lose their balance. I believe this effect is most pronounced when you see a child running—you can tell they are not relaxed and will not run at full speed. They're playing it safe because their brain is having trouble processing the conflicting information it's receiving.

Dyspraxia is another type of motion disorder that makes it hard to plan and coordinate physical movement. People with dyspraxia may not have balance issues but can experience difficulty executing simple tasks like turning a doorknob or brushing their teeth. It can even affect their ability to speak—in a way that's different than what was mentioned in the speech disorder chapter. This is not due to any muscle weakness but communication problems within the brain.

I believe dyspraxia is due to a problem in the thalamus, a part of your brain through which all sensory information routes.[i] When you move your arm to pick up a glass, there are two separate systems at work. The motor nerves in your arm are firing off commands to flex your muscles in such a way to pick up a glass. But just flexing a muscle is a very inaccurate way of moving parts of your body—you need feedback from your body to detect how far you've actually moved. Even with your eyes closed, you can reach your hand out in front of you and have a very good idea as to its position in space. This is not because your brain has kept a record of how many "move" commands it sent your arm, but because many muscles and tendons contain sensory receptors and can relay the precise amount of stretching they are experiencing.

With this incredible system working correctly, your brain will fire and receive thousands of commands to move and correct, move and correct—any time motion is required. When your thalamus is not working, it cannot process the sensory information properly and as a result, the "move and correct" sequence is disrupted. You can activate your muscles properly, but without any positional feedback, accurate movement becomes difficult. With effort, you can get your hands or mouth and tongue to do what you want them to do, but it does not happen easily and requires a considerable amount of concentration.

Luckily, many children outgrow this issue just like they might a crooked smile. It can be a subtle effect that makes them feel naturally uncoordinated, but there may be a lesion or inflammation causing the problem.

---

i. With some forms of dyspraxia there appears to be another cognitive issue that affects planning and initiation of movement.

EATING DISORDERS

Food aversion, taste sensitivities

The next time you happen to have cooked apples and cooked potatoes in front of you, close your eyes, pinch your nose and eat one of them at random. See if you can tell the difference. Most people don't realize how much your sense of smell contributes to taste.

A popular biochemist who crafted perfumes in Paris for many years said that smell is possible because a bit of your brain is exposed to the air inside your nose. Out of all the senses, the olfactory organ is thought to have the most intimate relationship with the brain—more so than sight or hearing or taste. This might explain why smells can often conjure up detailed memories of events long ago.

For me, I have a smell that is as close to time travel as any technology I've ever experienced. If I ever smell a plain saltine cracker, it is like magic. It takes me back to the nursery at the church I grew up in. I can feel myself opening the plastic jar the crackers were kept in. I can see the old green carpet and the portraits hanging on the wall. I can hear the little colored xylophone play itself as its dragged along the floor. I don't have to eat the cracker—just smell it. In fact, I can even think about the smell of a saltine cracker and experience some of these things.

I've spoken to many people who can identify a particular cleaning solution from their elementary school days. Though they wouldn't know what it looked like, or what is was called, a whiff of that same scent can instantly transport them decades in time to their childhood. Certain music has always had a similar effect on me, but it has never come close to the trip a smell might send me on.

The cranial nerves are numbered from one to twelve, in order from the front to the back. The cranial nerves at the front are closest to many other components of your brain, like the *Amygdala* and *Hippocampus*, where new memories are processed for long-term storage. Perhaps it's no coincidence that the 1st cranial nerve is the Olfactory nerve, and is responsible for conveying smells into your brain.

Because your sense of taste is affected by your nose as much as your tongue, problems with multiple cranial nerves can cause sensitivities to food—not in the allergic sense, but in a way that anything beyond bland feels like too much. While issues with the 1st cranial nerve may cause sensitivity to smell, issues with the 7th and 9th cranial nerves might cause hypersensitivity to taste. The 7th cranial nerve is responsible for moving the muscles on your face, but also receives input from the front two-thirds of your tongue. The 9th cranial nerve receives input from the back one-third of your tongue.

Food aversion is not as simple as taste preferences—cravings for carb-heavy diets might be a result of dysfunction within the area postrema.[85] Cancer patients can develop severe aversions to food consumed during nausea-inducing chemotherapy. More importantly, there can be a fear-driven response to certain foods that may seem unexplainable to the outside observer but is a primal survival response the person doing the eating has little control over. In illustrating his

Polyvagal Theory, Dr. Porges describes it in a way that reminds me of other fear responses:

> *"Taste aversion produces a regurgitative response that has adaptive function following the ingestion of contaminated foods. Taste aversion, similar to immobilization and dissociation, attempts to minimize life threat and internal injury."*[86]

For a child who has experienced immobilization and dissociation stressors, and who may be experiencing crippling anxiety, taste sensitivities may not even be necessary to create problems with eating. There can be multiple components to this, but as someone who has experienced food aversion my entire life, I can attest it is not an easy thing to overcome.

Latching issues, mastication problems

I have heard of mothers who were in the hospital with a baby that was latching on to their breast perfectly, only to find it suddenly developed problems once they got home. A lactation consultant may be called in for assistance, but after trying many different things, they are just not able to help. A bottle is tried without success. The mother may cycle through every variety of nipple available until finally—a particular shape seems to work. The baby is able to latch and eat again. If you have experienced an hours or day old infant suddenly not be able to eat, it can be a traumatic experience.

The same cranial nerves that can cause issues with speaking can also cause issues with eating. The 12th cranial nerve controls the majority of the tongue muscles and allows it to form different shapes required for speaking. Proper tongue control is also needed for latching, and a baby who is experiencing even partial paralysis may be unable to.

If a baby could latch perfectly and suddenly develops a problem—

this points to a 12th cranial nerve palsy. Unfortunately, the hepatitis B vaccine some infants receive at birth contains aluminum—easily enough to cause a 12th cranial nerve lesion and trigger this effect. Thankfully, most countries do not recommend administering the hepatitis B vaccine to infants and latching is not a problem. If you live in a country where this vaccine is suggested for your infant, you may want to consider waiting.

As your child grows older, the tongue serves another purpose in eating—mastication. As food is chewed in your mouth, the tongue is vital in positioning and rotating things in order that your teeth are able to break it down properly before it enters your stomach. If your child is old enough to eat solid foods that require mastication, they may have difficulty breaking down the food properly before they swallow. This phenomenon is not likely to happen without the accompaniment of a tongue-related speech disorder, but is something to watch out for.

Swallowing Problems

Probably the most common problems associated with eating is with difficulty in swallowing. The complex sequence of events that allow you to properly close the windpipe leading into your lungs and push food or liquid into your stomach requires the coordination of up to six cranial nerves.

Without going into a lengthy explanation of this process, the two that may cause the most problems are with the 9th and 10th cranial nerves. When food hits the back of your throat—the *pharynx*—it is supposed to initiate the beginning of the involuntary part of swallowing. If there is a problem with the 9th cranial nerve, it may not sense this event and consequentially, your swallow reflex is never even started. This phenomenon will be more evident with liquids as they do not create enough pressure on the pharynx to trigger the reflex.

If the 10th cranial nerves are not functioning properly, portions of the muscle constriction that actually push food downwards may not work. I've heard someone describe this as "throat freeze." They are mentally prepared to swallow their food, but fear creeps in as they know the muscles required to do it are not likely to cooperate.

Both 9th and 10th cranial nerves play a part in closing the windpipe during the swallow reflex. If this sequence is not happening properly, *aspiration* can happen—food or liquid can get into your lungs and can lead to numerous problems such as pneumonia.

Any of these issues can create crippling anxiety around eating. The person may be starving and completely enjoy the food they have been prepared, but if they cannot swallow it without fear of gagging or choking, they will often go hungry and begin to lose weight.

Indigestion, heartburn and acid reflux

Indigestion, heartburn, and acid reflux are three painful symptoms people with or without chronic infections can experience. The market for acid-suppressing drugs is massive and those who sell these products may not want you to realize a little secret about this problem—you have been told you have too much stomach acid when more often than not, the problem is actually too little.

Long-term stress and infections with bacteria like *H. Pylori* can cause a deficit in hydrochloric acid production. When the stomach doesn't have enough acid, food sits and putrefies instead of breaking down and moving on. In addition to breaking down the food, the stomach was made to be acidic in order to help "sterilize" food. As a result, the lining of the stomach constantly replaces itself in order to withstand the extremely low pH levels inside.[i] When the proper acid level is reached, the body will signal that the food is safe to pass into your intestines by opening the *pyloric valve* at the base of your stomach.

If there is not enough acid, this signal won't happen and the pyloric

---

i. Refresher: Low pH is more acidic.

valve won't open. As pressure builds inside, it will eventually be released through the upper stomach valve. With the upper valve open and you laying horizontally instead of standing upright, acid may come up, burning the inside of your esophagus. This is why medicines work —they reduce the acid so much that even when pressure builds to this point, there is not enough to reach your esophagus. They come with a price due to the fact your food is not being digested properly.

Obesity

It is not uncommon to see a child who appears much heavier than they should be. The immediate response may be to question the abilities of their parents to manage their health or discipline their food intake. You might see a severely overweight child amongst their family, none of whom appear to have weight issues, and wonder what their problem is.

You may have one of these children, who for no apparent reason is much heavier than their siblings. Some of them may seem to have a voracious appetite that can never be satisfied, while others consume similar amounts of food as their siblings but put on weight at a rate that doesn't seem right.

While healthy eating and exercise are certainly important habits for every child (and parent) to master, many see their child's weight balloon in a way that is clearly unnatural. Before you beat yourself—or someone else—up about being a horrible parent, either of these scenarios may be explained by a physiological dysfunction.

Thyroid problems are not normally associated with children, but should still be ruled out. The markers for hypothyroidism are not always clear, but care should be taken to ensure a child is not putting on weight because of too little thyroid hormone in their body. This may occasionally be the issue, but I believe another problem is more commonly the cause.

The hypothalamus is an important area of your brain that controls, among other things, hunger. There are three separate areas that coordinate responses within your body to recognize the physical feeling of fullness They read the chemical clues your body creates to indicate it needs more food and issue signals that you need to eat. Chronic inflammation or lesions from metal toxicity can disrupt this sophisticated process, creating a seemingly insatiable hunger that is never satisfied. This might be purely because the physical sensors in your stomach that signal it is full are not being interpreted correctly, or because your hypothalamus is issuing commands to eat even though the rest of your body is not requesting it.

This may seem like a scientific stretch to justify the poor eating habits of an undisciplined kid, but in animal models, scientists can purposefully induce a lesion in a specific region the hypothalamus and create obesity. If your child has no thyroid issue and seems to always want to eat, you may want to think about treating them for metal toxicity or chronic inflammation that may be causing it.

Anorexia

In the same way that scientists can create obesity by manipulating the hypothalamus, they can also create anorexia.[87] In mouse models, they can observe anorexia after damage to the hypothalamus.[88]

Anorexia is called *anorexia nervosa* because it was originally thought to be one of the many diseases of the nervous system—a part of *neurasthenia*, or what I believe we would have called autoimmune disorders. Though these studies mention their ability to create anorexia, they are actually only creating a portion of anorexia—the intense food aversion that causes weight loss. People who experience anorexia have many other symptoms that are not specifically related to food such as extreme anxiety, which can be triggered by a dysfunctional hypothalamic-pituitary axis, and OCD behaviors, which can be triggered by problems with a neighboring organ—the thalamus.

The complexities of anorexia nervosa might require several chapters to explore, but I wanted to mention these three phenomena together—extreme food aversion, anxiety and OCD—in case you might have noticed the sudden onset of these behaviors coinciding with an immune activation event such as stress or extreme physical exertion. I heard of a high school track team where three of the girls on the team developed anorexia within months of each other. Whether they'd been required to receive some shots to participate on the team, I cannot say, but it would certainly be unsurprising if they had. The combination of metal and microbes can do very strange things and while I might have once written off the coincidence, I now believe these three attributes may point to a common source.

BEHAVIORAL DISORDERS

In this chapter, I am going to go over some common behavioral issues you may have seen in your children (or yourself) and attempt to explain them in light of what I believe to be happening with metals, microbes and medicine. If you have seen a sudden change in behavior with your child that involves OCD tendencies, destructive behaviors, hurting themselves or epic meltdowns, take a look at the chapter on PANDAS/PANS—it might explain what your child is going through.

OCD (lining up toys, problems with changes in plans)

Some children may have extremely heightened anxiety and an exaggerated fight or flight response profile. This may be due to problems with the vagal system and the way it communicates information to various hormone producing organs around the body. It can also be due to a dysfunctioning hypothalamus or even possibly trauma. For children that are in a state of chronic hyper-arousal, novel stimuli can be interpreted as a potential threat. This is why some children react so strongly against change—in their heightened state of arousal, the smallest adjustment might feel similar to a hidden animal suddenly charging at them from out of nowhere—the equivalent of a life-threatening situation.

Although it may sound absurd, this kind of elevated fight or flight response can permeate into every event of the day. Parents who could not find their children's favorite socks to wear and had to cancel dinner plans because of it will be able to relate. Humans are naturally exploratory creatures but to children who are in a state of hyper-arousal and are unsure of what is friend or foe, anything new can generate extreme anxiety.

You have probably seen pictures, if not experienced it yourself, of children lining up cars, toys, blocks—nearly anything—for an hour at a time. While other children may be making engine noises and directing toy cars all over the living room furniture in a wonderful display of imagination, you will often see children with other signs of autism stacking, sorting and ordering.

"Superior pattern matching is the essence of the evolved brain…"[89] according to a 2014 study published in Frontiers of Neuroscience. Pattern matching is the foundation of the decision making strategies we develop as infants and may use until our last day on earth. Other animals use pattern-matching. Many birds may use it for their uncanny navigational abilities that allow them to find their nest in someone's backyard, even though they were blindfolded and transported hundreds of miles away in a car.

Children with autism may have deficits in certain types of pattern matching. As the 2014 paper put it:

"the ability to predict the thought processes and actions of others provides major advantages in navigating what are often complex social landscapes in human societies. However, the inferring of agency, beliefs and intentions in others, is dysregulated in… autism spectrum disorders."

At the same time, they may excel in other areas, such as abilities required to understand music or spatial pattern matching. Novelty exploration inevitably requires risk, and in the hyper-aroused child, a novel experience may present tremendous anxiety. Children in this state may exhibit strange play with toys not because they are incapable of imagining that a car could jump over the magazines on the coffee table, but because they are afraid to try. Once the initial enjoyment of pattern-matching has been discovered, probably by complete accident, many children may find that employing their abilities by ordering and sorting things makes them feel much safer and more calm than the unknowns of imaginative play.

While their constant repetition and apparent lack of imagination may make you feel that they aren't growing, they are likely exploring new pattern creation you may not be able to detect: Color sorting by saturation rather than hue. By weight. By order in which they first played each toy. By smell. There are a thousand patterns that may exist beyond our awareness when your "superior pattern matching" is focused in one area.

Hand flapping and finger snapping –

It is my suspicion that lesions in the 10th cranial nerve nuclei or the hypothalamic-pituitary axis (HPA) can create the inappropriate release of epinephrine (adrenaline) or cortisol. The vagus nerve normally works to control the body's natural response to fear and excitement. If it's not working correctly, even mild stimuli can create hyper-arousal. Problems with cranial nerve dysfunction or the HPA could cause anxiety and trigger physical behaviors designed to restore the hormone imbalance.

When humans get extremely excited, whether out of fear or joy, they move their bodies. Whether cavemen were giving each other high-fives is up for debate but throwing one's arms up in the air in celebration is a primal instinct that never needs to be taught—as natural as covering your mouth when witnessing something horrible.

Although a quick shot of cortisol could help save your life in times of stress, your body doesn't like the way it feels: an upset stomach, extreme anxiety, jitters, difficulty sleeping, a suppressed immune response. Instinctively, your body knows that elevated levels of cortisol are not good for it—so it tries to get rid of it.

Physical activity is the simplest way your body can "burn off" cortisol. When it senses there is too much, you may find yourself pacing or if sitting – bouncing your legs. When children, who lack the self-awareness of adults, have elevated cortisol levels, they do what their body tells them to do to get rid of it—they shake their arms, flap their hands, or snap their fingers.

I have seen videos of young babies—not old enough to even turn over onto their stomach—flapping their hands. This can be a natural attempt at restoring the hormonal imbalance that excitement causes, such as hearing a favorite song or seeing their favorite cartoon character. If the flapping continues unabated, even in the absence of such stimuli, I would begin to suspect they are instinctively trying to get rid of the inappropriate amounts of cortisol or adrenaline their body is producing.

Behavioral specialists may tell you they are doing this because it makes them feel good, but in prolonged flapping sequences with no stimuli to explain it, I believe they are doing it because it makes them feel *better*, not good. As a parent, I realize this is a horrible thing to hear about your child. You want so badly to help them, and any of these little signs of anxiety or stress can be so difficult to deal with.

Destructive behavior (tantrums, screaming, head banging,

scratching, cutting and burning)

Destructive behaviors are often an inappropriate attempt at defusing the acute anxiety someone may be experiencing. In children with extremely elevated levels of norepinephrine or cortisol, their body is primed for battle or escape. In a typical human, if the battle or escape attempt doesn't happen, their stress hormones should eventually return back to normal levels, allowing their gut and immune system to begin working at full strength again. In someone with acute anxiety from problems in their hypothalamic-pituitary axis or locus coeruleus, the hormones never return to an appropriate level. Their body can sense this is unhealthy and will essentially simulate the fight or flight response to use up the excess stress hormones.

This means you will see the fight—hitting siblings or parents, throwing chairs or food to the ground, slamming doors—any physical action they can to use up the excess epinephrine or cortisol. Similarly, you will hear all the primal utterances anyone in a fight for their life might make—screaming, crying, and taunts. Certain children will exhibit the flight behavior—they will run away, as fast as they can. You are not the perceived threat in this scenario—there is none. But their body is telling them otherwise and is doing everything it can to bring back the appropriate chemistry.

This behavior is absolutely horrifying to watch, but for a confused child whose body is signaling to them the state they are in is extremely unhealthy, it may just be an attempt to correct itself through these destructive behaviors. As the child matures, they will be disciplined for these outbursts and will feel they have no outlet through which to defuse their anxiety. I believe it is these children that resort to self-injurious behaviors such as clawing at their face or hitting their heads against the wall. They are old enough to understand that destroying things or screaming is unacceptable but have no other way to channel their excess "fight." So they hurt themselves, because they know that hurting others or throwing fits is wrong.

Watching someone hurt themselves is probably one of the most traumatic things someone can witness. As they get older, those especially affected may resort to cutting themselves with knives or razor blades, even burning themselves with candles or cigarettes. Components of anorexia nervosa seem to fall under this umbrella. Besides having a complete unwillingness to eat, they will often exhibit self-injurious behaviors.

A dysfunctional immune system may explain this behavior. If you have ever had a crushing headache, you may have felt compelled to bang your head against a solid object. What would cause this seemingly counterintuitive, instinctual response? I believe our bodies intuit the healing response of the immune system and can sense when it's not working.

After inflammation comes healing, and our bodies are intimately familiar with this sequence. When there is pain in the body and healing does not come, our brain senses the healing process is not working. It responds by creating more inflammation—more pain—because that is what triggers the immune response. If your body does not appear to be addressing the crippling headache you are experiencing, then perhaps it didn't get the message. Instinctively, you create additional inflammation by banging your head against a wall. Although the temporary pain is immense and worse than it already was, it is done in the desperate hope that this time your body will respond to the request for help.

I believe this particular behavior may be a clear indication of a critically depressed immune system—your body can sense that the normal immune response that accompanies pain is not responding to its requests. In a severely dysfunctional immune system flush with chronic infection, the signals may not get sent at all. So your body instinctively tries to generate a crystal clear message to your immune system—send help here now.

POTS

POTS is a rare disease that affects men and women and is most commonly diagnosed because of an abnormal heart beat upon standing. If you've ever been lying down, stood up suddenly, then experienced faintness or dizziness, imagine a much more severe form of that feeling created just by standing slowly—possibly even simply by sitting up. Seconds, then minutes pass by, but the disorientation and fluttering heart remain. For some, lying down is the only thing that can ease the symptoms. As doctors struggle to diagnose the problem, children might have to drop out of school and adults sometimes must quit their job.

The onset of POTS, like many of the illnesses discussed in this book, is associated with an infection, pregnancy or surgery. People that have developed problems after the Gardasil vaccine are often diagnosed with this illness.[90] And like many of the modern illnesses, its symptoms are so varied as to make you wonder where one disease starts and the other stops.

A procedure specialists can use to diagnose POTS is called a tilt table test. The patient lies down flat on a table and is observed with a blood pressure monitor and electrocardiography. After their baseline measurements are taken, the table will tilt into more of a vertical position and their measurements will be taken again. Some tests can measure blood pressure in multiple areas of the body, such as the lower legs, chest and head to compare the differences. If the patient shows significant differentials in blood pressure between the two tilting positions, it indicates they may have the condition.

A quick look through a "Living with POTS" website shows a young girl, struggling to deal with the effects of the disorder. Her picture shows unmistakable left side facial palsy—up on the right, down on the left. Her condition initially gave her terrible anxiety and she would routinely have panic attacks. She provides another interesting detail: she has become extremely sound sensitive and doesn't like going to places because of it. She can't go to movies, malls or even church because of the noise.

Currently, the cause of POTS is considered unknown. I'd like to explain two things: the mechanism causing POTS symptoms, and the reasons these mechanisms are happening.

If you've ever flown in a fighter jet or an airplane capable of creating extreme g-forces, you will have worn a special outfit called a G-suit. The purpose of this device is to prevent blood from pooling in your legs during a high-speed maneuver. The suit is connected to the flight controls of the plane and will automatically force air into bladders around your legs and abdomen as needed—the more extreme the maneuver, the tighter the suit will squeeze around your body.

Without this suit, the centrifugal forces would push the blood in your head down as far as possible into your body. Your feet and legs would swell with incredible pressure as your brain developed *hypoxia* from a lack of oxygen. Your vision would become progressively foggier until you lost consciousness. If you've ever ridden on a roller coaster where your feet hang freely under the ride, you will have experienced a mild form of this at the bottom of hills and at the top of loops as blood is driven into your legs.

Although this may seem like an extreme example, the G-suit that allows pilots to perform extended high-speed maneuvers is based on a design we all already have in our bodies called *vasoconstriction*. Without consciously thinking about it, your body is constantly adjusting the muscular walls around the arteries as you change positions. When you are standing, the weight of all the blood in your body will tend to push down into your feet and legs. To counter this, your body squeezes the arteries in your legs to make them smaller, forcing more of the blood to stay in your head. When you lay down, this additional pressure isn't needed, and the muscles around the arteries in your legs relax, allowing the blood to flow freely throughout your body.

With POTS, the vasoconstriction that happens automatically is not working. Your body does not respond to positional changes and as such, the blood pools in your legs and feet when you stand or sit. You will experience the effects of not enough oxygen in your brain—dizziness, headaches, brain fog, and many other issues. Your heart will sense a drop in blood pressure and try to compensate by speeding up.

This is why IV fluids can be a godsend for people suffering with POTS. The added saline creates an artificial rise in blood pressure that offsets the drop from standing. The blood will still pool in your legs inappropriately, but with the added volume of blood, it doesn't affect you as much.

If you or someone you love is suffering from POTS, it may feel like a mysterious and complicated disorder. I think it actually has a very simple cause—which means it may have a very simple fix.

⚹ ⚹ ⚹

Several sensors in your body called *baroreceptors* detect changes in your blood pressure. They wrap around blood vessels and are activated when they are shortened or stretched. If you stand up, blood flows down into your body causing the vessels in the carotid artery in your neck to shrink. Your body senses this immediately and sends out commands to constrict the blood vessels in your legs. Just like the pilot's G-suit, your legs adjust for this drop in blood pressure to make it easier to keep the brain functioning properly. It may also raise the heart rate to compensate.

Another reflex called the *vestibulosympathetic reflex* conveys changes in posture and orientation in order that the body can make blood pressure and heart rate adjustments.[91] This reflex happens through the 8th cranial nerve and is combined with pressure change information received from the baroreceptors around the body in the *solitary nucleus*. The solitary nucleus is an area of your brain stem that just happens to be millimeters away from many of the other cranial nerve nuclei that seem to develop problems so often.

When this information is properly interpreted, the brain will issue commands to increase the heart rate and make adjustments to the *vasoconstriction* of various blood vessels around the body. If this information is not received or conveyed properly, there will be problems associated with POTS.

The 8th cranial nerve is called the vestibulocochlear nerve and is responsible for hearing and movement. You may remember that the girl in the story above had developed extreme sound sensitivity. This actually has nothing to do with the 8th cranial nerve but is due to a 7th cranial nerve palsy—something we can easily detect that she has by the picture on the website. The 7th cranial nerve innervates the tiniest muscle in your body—the stapedius muscle. This muscle is used to control a bone that dampens loud noises in your ear, and when it's not working correctly, things sound very loud.

If someone has developed a lesion in the solitary nucleus, they will have difficulty sensing inputs from changes in blood pressure correctly. Similarly, if they develop a lesion in the 8th cranial nerve, they may have difficulty sending the correct postural and orientation change information to the brain. Problems with either of these inputs could cause the symptoms of POTS.

If it is a 8th cranial nerve problem, they are likely to have other motion disorder issues, such as vertigo, nystagmus, or dyspraxia. With this particular problem, their heart and blood pressure may have trouble adjusting to changes in body position, but will eventually correct itself.

If they have a lesion in the solitary nucleus, their body will not make the changes required to maintain proper blood pressure and flow, no matter how long they stand. If they are someone who tends to have low blood pressure to begin with, they may have trouble even sitting.

If they have a problem with their vagal system, it may not be able to properly convey messages about raising the heart rate or constricting the blood vessels in the legs. If they have other issues associated with vagus nerve dysfunction such as *gastroparesis*[i], constipation, or extreme anxiety, we may assume that is where the problem lies.

I have heard of people with POTS who have developed crippling headaches, sometimes strange headaches that wrap around the back of their head "like the legs of a spider." These headaches seem to be on the surface of the head as much as inside and could be caused by lesions on the *occipital* and *auricular nerves*.

These nerves wrap around the back and sides of your head and originate an inch or so away from the solitary nucleus, the area of your brain stem where I believe most POTS dysfunction is caused. I have covered this elsewhere, but where motor neuron lesions tend to cause

---

i. A condition that affects the stomach muscles and prevents proper stomach emptying.

weakness, sensory nerve lesions tend to cause extreme sensitivity, even pain.

If aluminum is damaging this area of the brain, it would make sense that blood pressure and heart rate problems would often coincide with anxiety issues, gut issues and strange headaches. In fact, this area of the brain is so tightly packed, it would be extremely unlikely to experience only one of these symptoms.

POTS is most likely caused by lesions in the solitary nucleus in the brainstem—lesions which are most likely caused by aluminum.[ii] As horrible as the disease is, it is the same exact thing that causes crooked smiles and misaligned eyes. If you spot someone with a crooked face and they are otherwise fine, just remember the difference a millimeter or two could make.

---

ii. This is probably why the Gardasil vaccine is commonly associated with POTS and some of these other issues—it easily contains enough aluminum hydroxide to cause these lesions.

TICS, TOURETTE'S & FACIAL PAIN

TIC-DOULOUREUX. (1837)
CASE 1.
A Lady fifty-five years of age has been affected for the last thirty-six years with tic-douloureux in the cheek, and in the forehead above the eyebrow, on the left side … Her sufferings during the continuance have been extreme, and have compelled her to confine herself to bed until its termination, and it has never lasted a shorter time than two days… She had a paralytic affection of the elevator muscle of the upper eyelid, and of the left side of the face. Morphia, strychnine, and other means had been used to a great extent, but without any other effect than to induce debility…[92]

CASE 2
Mr. C., aged forty, has laboured for sixteen years under tic-douloureux over the right side of the face and forehead, but particularly along the lower jaw as far as the chin… During the whole course of the disease, this patient has rarely been free

from pain… He had taken large doses of carbonate of iron, arsenic, mercury, opium, morphia … without effect; and when he came under treatment … he was directed to take small doses of blue pill with Epsom salts… Soon after this, he gave up the use of the internal medicines, and gradually improved under the influence of the Veratria alone; the intervals became longer, and the fits less and less painful, until at the end of four weeks from the time he came under treatment, he returned home perfectly free from pain.[93]

CASE 3

A Lady, forty-eight years with tic-douloureux, situated in the left side of the face, for a period of twenty-two years. She has made use of a variety of medicines, particularly carbonate of iron, which she had taken for three months in very large doses, but without experiencing any benefit… A short time before this patient came under treatment she had an attack of paralysis from which she had recovered, with the exception of a slight palsied appearance of the countenance.[94]

As surgeons in the early 1800s advanced their understanding of the nervous system, people began to seek treatment for a mysterious illness they called *tic douloureux*—often experienced as a horrible stabbing pain in one side of the face. The attacks could be sudden and so intense their face would involuntarily twitch. Like nearly any illness of the day, it was often attributed to problems in the gut, and so copious amounts of mercuric medicine were administered to purge the intestines. If this didn't work, surgeons might sever the 5th cranial nerve in an often futile attempt to end their agonizing suffering.

Both modern doctors and people currently suffering from unexplained facial pain seem unaware of the terrible history of tic douloureux. It is now called *persistent idiopathic facial pain* after having been referred to as *atypical facial pain* for many years.

After reading through early accounts of this disorder, you will notice many of the same patterns we see in other diseases that appeared *en masse* around this same time period. One—the onset of the disease was preceded by another, more trivial illness that was treated with metallic medicines. Two—the patients often experienced facial palsy alongside whatever the illness might be. Three—the mysterious disease (and sometimes the facial palsy) disappeared once the metallic medicines stopped being administered.

It is difficult to read these accounts of suffering, hundreds of years old though they may be, and not shake your fists at the obviousness the patients and their doctors were missing. The environmental ingestion of metals through Paris Green[i] might have played a big part in their maladies, but the medicines they were being administered with every cough and sneeze contained enough neurotoxins to kill someone.

It is no wonder the mortality of nearly every disease on the planet plummeted towards the end of the 1800s when the use of metals as medicine began to decline. The fact that many of these people showed the signs of metal poisoning on their faces should reinforce the theory that crooked faces serve as warning signs to the toxicity of our modern-day metallic medicines.

I mention it in the chapter on Behavioral Disorders but wanted to leave the thought here as well in case it rings true. You may notice your infant spontaneously scream out in pain. Not a sustained scream that is sometimes associated with *encephalopathy* or the semi-sustained cries of a baby with bowel issues. I'm referring to a sudden shriek. You will notice it because it doesn't feel like a vocal experimentation, but an expression of pain. These are horrible outbursts to witness as a parent and often there appears to be no cause.

---

i. Arsenic is considered a metalloid rather than a metal, a distinction too subtle to keep mentioning directly within the text.

After having read of the accounts of the suffering of people from two hundred years ago with tic douloureux—and seeing the contortions visible on a baby's face—I cannot help but to wonder if they may be suffering the effects of 5th cranial nerve palsy. Idiopathic, according to the doctors—an unknown cause. But perhaps we can understand why.

What causes facial tics?

It is my theory that for some people, a component of tics—the little twitches and spasms you often see on people's faces—are "tic douloureux-lite", a subtle, almost painless form of the same 5th cranial nerve palsy that causes the unexplainable facial pain some people develop. This would suggest that tics are not *motor* disorders, but are in fact *sensory* disorders.

Much like a horse twitches their skin when they sense a fly may have landed on their back, the 7th cranial nerve may twitch the face—if the 5th cranial nerve mistakenly signals to the brain something significant happened. Whether there was actually pain or not does not matter—your brain will automatically process the input and send the response down the 7th cranial nerve to act. Your cheek, or forehead or eyelid or mouth will scrunch or twist involuntarily and you will demonstrate what we call facial tics.

Sometimes the 5th cranial nerve will both generate the phantom pain signal and receive the response for movement—you will see this displayed by someone "popping" their jaw, a common facial tic. Though I point to the pattern of sensory hyper-activity and motor under-activity, a dysfunctioning 11th cranial nerve (which controls neck and shoulder muscles) could be the cause of the frequent head snaps and shoulder shrugs seen with Tourette syndrome.

What about vocal tics?

The 10th cranial nerve is responsible for the enervation of the vocal chords. This makes me wonder if vocal tics are simply "unvoluntary"[i] vocalizations (caused by a dysfunctioning 10th cranial nerve) that are channeled into actual words and phrases. Most of us respond to pain with the word "Ouch!" It is an instinctual response that happens instantly, without a millisecond of thought as to what to say. Some of us may function at a higher level and actually have two choices—"Ouch" or "Shit"—depending on the context. In this case, in a situation of extreme pain or anxiety, our control over that decision may not happen consciously and we may say something we didn't intend.

I believe a part of this same phenomenon is occurring with vocal tics. Because speaking is such a primal human instinct, perhaps the embarrassment of what would have been a spontaneous grunt or squeak is lessened by forming it into an intelligible word—a word or set of words that the brain, in its mysterious ways, associates and locks in to a particular tic.

This effect would happen so quickly that the speaker would not be conscious of having made a word choice—just like they have no control over their sound choices. They might have consciously done it the first or second time, as is evidenced by the apparent "contagiousness" of vocal tics when people with Tourette syndrome gather. But after that first semi-conscious choice, the brain locks the pattern in, just as it has with "Ouch." This also might explain why younger children with Tourette syndrome emit more squeaks and pips, while older people tend towards actual words.

What about tics that involve hands and upper body?

Not all tics are due to cranial nerve palsies. Inflammation in the

---

i. The word unvoluntary is used instead of involuntary on purpose. Unvoluntary actions can be suppressed, to an extent. Involuntary actions cannot.

thalamus and other parts of the brain can trigger these movements. It could also trigger phantom pain internally, causing the full body movements that some people experience.

The reasons behind tics and Tourette syndrome are poorly understood and obviously can't be explained by phantom pains created by dysfunctional nerves alone. However, I do believe there is a connection. A glimpse through videos of people bravely demonstrating their various tics will frequently reveal signs of other cranial nerve palsies—partial eye blinks, asymmetrical smiles and misaligned eyes— a sign to me of cranial nerve dysfunction.

After having read about tic douloureux appearing alongside the administration of metal as medicine, I can't help but to wonder if the modern-day version—tics and Tourette syndrome—are caused by the same thing.

A VERY EARLY CASE OF AUTISM?

The current DSM-5 diagnosis for autism focuses on two things. The first is "Persistent deficits in social communication and social interaction across multiple contexts…"[95] The other is "Restricted, repetitive patterns of behavior, interests, or activities…" For all the varied neurological symptoms and behaviors we see in children nowadays, coming up with a universal set of diagnostic criteria that describes each and every child is difficult. These two do a good job of describing the most common traits, but there are other common symptoms that frequently appear alongside: Bowel disorders.[i] Anxiety and behavioral issues. Sensory disorders. Sometimes incredible artistic gifts.

Although the DSM-5 diagnosis is a good general description of autism, most children with the disorder exhibit one or more of what I will refer to as *secondary traits*. The *primary traits* are those described by the DSM-5: social deficits and repetitive behaviors. The secondary

---

i. A benign exploration of this association in the late 1990s would cause minor troubles for a British gastroenterologist.

traits are more varied, but ultimately can cause more suffering than problems with social integration and OCD-like behaviors which define the disorder.

Autism, as we now know it, does not appear to exist in the medical literature before Leo Kanner's original account, "Autistic disturbances of effective contact" was released in April of 1943. He had just published a 527-page textbook called "Child Psychiatry" eight years earlier, and the massive tome contained nothing resembling this new disorder—despite covering obscure psychiatric illnesses most people would not recognize. This is not to say autism did not exist, but if it did, was so rare that it doesn't appear in the medical literature. However, glimpses of it, particularly some of the secondary traits that often accompany autism diagnoses are clearly visible if you look closely.

Amongst the other cases Bell presented are a few curious accounts, one of which is particularly interesting because of its striking similarity to someone we might think of as autistic.

No. XVII

Francis Robbins, æt. 19, has been short-sighted from his infancy. The structure of the eyes appears perfectly natural. The pupils are less contracted by the application of a strong light than is usual. I have seen him frequently during the last six or seven years, and have always observed that the eye-balls are in constant motion, not upwards and downwards, but laterally. He is of a very nervous temperament, and upon the slightest excitement this motion of the eyes is considerably increased, and no effort to look steadily at an object placed before him has any effect in restraining it. His vision does not deceive him as to the state of things he looks at: he is sensible when objects are perfectly at rest, and perceives immediately the true direction of the slightest motion which is given to them: he can read music with facility, and plays accurately from the notes rapid passages on the violin. If he is surrounded by many moving objects his vision becomes confused, and he forms an erroneous judgment as to their distance from each other, and from himself. Thus, in the morning early, before the streets are crowded, he drives a carriage and pair of horses with safety and dexterity, but he cannot do this in the middle of the day, when, to use his own expression, "he gets flustered" and is afraid of meeting with accidents.[96]

From the very beginning, mention of his dilated, uncooperative pupils should throw up a red flag for anyone who has studied metal toxicity. Secondly, he is obviously displaying signs of *nystagmus*, a quick, often lateral flicking of the eyes. Amongst other vision problems, nystagmus is a common secondary trait in autism.[97] Anxiety disorders are another common secondary trait in children on the autism spectrum,[98] and hearing a 19-year-old man described as having "a very nervous temperament" strikes me as out of the ordinary. Bell is surprised at the visual acuity that the teen displays, despite the abnormal eye movements. The comment that he "perceives immediately the true direction of the slightest motion…" also stands out as a common secondary trait of autism. Researchers have noticed this phenomenon and have tried to understand why kids with autism can detect motion sometimes twice as fast as their peers.[99] His apparent musical giftedness will be no surprise to many parents of autistic children,[100] and finally, his difficulty in coping with large crowds sounds familiar. Perhaps it's related to his vision problems, but getting "flustered" amidst the noise of a crowded city street would not be out of place with an autistic child, no matter the reason.

Could this young man be an early account of someone with signs of acute metal toxicity we might today call autism? Unfortunately, we don't have enough information to determine if he had deficits in social communication or interaction, and there are no signs of repetitive behavior. However, the secondary traits (and hints to possible metal toxicity) are unmistakable to me.

I propose that the "primary" traits of autism, those first two criteria listed in the DSM-5 handbook, are the result of fetal and infant exposure to metals, which are in turn causing chronic immune activation that cripple the developing brain. The other "secondary" traits that frequently go with autism—the gut issues, the vision problems, the anxiety, the behavioral problems and sensory disorders— those are caused by a different mechanism: acute damage from neurotoxins in the cranial nerves sometime after birth—often between the 12 and 18-month mark.

Chronic immune activation as a cause of the "primary" autistic traits is not a pet theory of mine, but is thoroughly supported by the most recent research available. It's a complex sequence of events that causes this, something well understood, and I will not attempt to explain it in this book. Others, such as Generation Rescue founder J.B. Handley, have done a much better job explaining this mechanism[101] than I could.[ii]

I propose the "secondary" traits are caused by a secondary assault upon a specific part of the brain, often a bit later in the child's life. Nearly any of the secondary traits of autism could be caused by damage to the various cranial nerves. Whereas the primary autistic traits are sometimes recognized slowly over time, the secondary traits often have an acute onset—these are the traits that parents frequently associate temporally with vaccination.

Why *this* specific part of the brain might be targeted by vaccines would become an obsession—a tangled riddle that would end with a possible answer that was more horrifying than anything I could have ever imagined.

---

ii. See endnote for a link explaining this entire chain of events.

THE DORSAL VAGAL COMPLEX

I had become familiar with the twelve cranial nerves and the effects their dysfunction could have on the human body, but wanted to understand why white blood cells carrying toxic metals might go there. If the aluminum was indeed being carried to specific places because of signaling from immune activation events, why the cranial nerves? Why was the immune system signaling for help into that specific area of the head?

As I looked through some 3-dimensional models of the human brain, something struck me—as I traced the routes of all the different cranial nerves I had been studying—the 7th, which made your smile crooked, the 3rd, 4th and 6th, which could cause your eyes to cross, and even the 8th, 9th and 10th cranial nerves—all of these fibers emerged from the same place on the brain stem. I immediately opened my anatomy book to look inside that section of the brain and found them labeled—the Pons and the Medulla Oblongata, primitive parts of the brain whose design is crucial to survival and is present even amongst reptiles.

All of the overlap I had been seeing—kids with Apraxia[i] who also showed 7th cranial nerve palsy, a woman with Dyspraxia[ii] who also showed 7th cranial nerve palsy, kids with autism who had strabismus caused by 3rd or 6th cranial nerve palsies, the babies with Torticollis that also showed 7th cranial nerve palsies of crooked smiles—amongst all these different people, with a constellation of various cranial nerve palsies, and now it made sense as to why. All of these palsies could easily have originated from the same place—a portion of the brain stem so small you could almost fit it inside a ping-pong ball.

An important area from which some of these cranial nerves originate has a special name, the *dorsal vagal complex*. This area of the brain stem includes the source of the 10th cranial nerve, the vagus nerve. Components of your brain inside this region control important parts of your *autonomic* nervous system, which functions to regulate your heart rate, your respiratory rate, and your intestines amongst a few others—all things which happen automatically, without you consciously thinking about it.

Besides the obvious function of your heart, digestion and breathing, the Dorsal Vagal Complex serves another important purpose—it works to mobilize your body should it sense danger. It can divert blood away from the gastrointestinal tract—even scavenging blood from just under the skin—and direct it to the skeletal muscles. It can prepare your lungs for increased efficiency. It can even increase your heart rate and dilate your eyes—all in preparation for dealing with an imminent threat.

There was something about this particular area and the cranial nerve nuclei that surround it that seemed to be damaged frequently. From crooked faces to the secondary traits of autism, if there were problems in someone that could be attributable to metal toxicity, there

---

i. Speech disorder
ii. Motion coordination disorder

was a good chance it originated here.

An obvious question began to form—the epicenter of our some of our most important cranial nerves appeared to be the site of frequent damage by the metals being injected into our body, but why?

If it was aluminum causing the damage, and the aluminum-containing white blood cells only traveled to specific places they were being signaled by your immune system—why the dorsal vagal complex? Why would the immune system signal for help there, out of all the places in your body?

Though I would eventually discover three reasons the immune system signals for help in the dorsal vagal complex, the first two came together when I was studying the role of the vagus nerve in the inflammatory system.[102]

The vagus nerve is about 20% motor nerves. The rest are sensory and spend all of their time receiving input from peripheral organs around the body. The information from these inputs is sent to specific cranial nerve nuclei within the brainstem for various reasons, most of which include important information about the status of your health.

A 2009 study demonstrated how chronic intestinal inflammation can negatively affect the neurons within the dorsal vagal complex.[103] A similar study[104] in 2003 showed significant activation of the brain's immune system, the microglia, after colitis was purposefully induced in the animals they were studying. Combined with the earlier study that recognized significant MCP-1 immune signaling *in the brain* after inflammation was produced in the liver,[105] this scientific research began to paint a clear picture of two ways in which the dorsal vagal complex can be immune activated: pathogen invasion and tissue injury.

Other studies[106][107] point to this specific trigger—something called the *inflammatory response*—a reflexive event that happens in a specific part of your brain whenever your body detects the invasion of a foreign invader or physical injury to your tissue.

Needless to say, I was stunned—both of these two triggers happen at the same time you get a shot. Pathogens invade your body, in the form of any viral or bacterial components of the vaccine, not to mention the other ingredients like aluminum or polysorbate 80. Most vaccines require an injection, something which would obviously be considered a tissue injury—minor perhaps compared to a stab wound or a dog bite, but still—both triggers are there, every time you get a shot.

The timing of it was what bothered me especially. Directly after an injection, the white blood cells which contain aluminum are floating freely around your body, ready to go wherever they are signaled. If the pathogen invasion and tissue injury were much later, that same aluminum would likely be less accessible inside muscle tissue or granulomas your body formed around them to protect itself.

As it so happens, vaccines are administered in such a way they cause both triggers for immune activation in the dorsal vagal complex —and many of them simultaneously introduce the very ingredient you wouldn't ever want to get transported into that area. It seemed like the perfect crime—as if someone had purposefully designed this event to cause neurological damage. After having seen the rise in childhood neurological disorders over the past twenty years, I couldn't believe they weren't higher.

When I learned that these two specific events were mentioned as immune activation triggers, the answer was clear—this was why the dorsal vagal complex was getting so much damage. This was why cranial nerve problems were so common. The crooked faces that I had noticed seemingly everywhere were most likely because the neurotoxin causing the cranial nerve lesions was introduced in such a way the body was practically begging for it to come wreck the part of your brain stem that controlled your face and your eyes. But other parts, too

—your intestines, your mood, your behavior and anxiety. Your ability to sleep well. Your ability to hear, taste, see and smell correctly. All of the illnesses associated with cranial nerves could be due to this one act —an injection of aluminum.

I thought back to the early cases of Charles Bell and the various cranial nerve palsies that started showing up in the early 1800s. They were receiving massive doses of mercury compared to the aluminum we were getting, but it was ingested, not injected. The body was able to filter most of it out. But the biggest difference was they were being administered the metals in pills and powders, often chased with a drink to hide its foul taste. They were not being injected.

They didn't have the pathogen invasion, and they didn't have the tissue injury. Unlike us, their dorsal vagal complex was not signaling for help from the white blood cells (which we assume would have contained mercury). They had so much metal toxicity it was inevitable cranial nerve damage would happen—possibly later on, during a sickness or after receiving some head injury. The resulting inflammation would have captured some of those white blood cells that contained mercury and generated the same effect—not just the crooked smiles and misaligned eyes, but all the other cranial nerve symptoms we see today.

The lack of pathogen invasion and tissue injury is why crooked faces are so seldom seen in the early daguerreotype and tin type images. The cranial nerve damage was there, but it was rare. It was the same cause—neurotoxins in the form of medicinal metals, but the inflammatory reflex that would signal the mercury towards the dorsal vagal complex was missing.

As I mentioned, there is a third reason the body creates immune activation within the dorsal vagal complex. This horrific discovery would haunt my attempts at sleep for days. If it turns out to be true, then we have a much bigger problem to deal with than I thought.

NEURASTHENIA & SHELL SHOCK

"Successfully leading men in war, like most work in life that does not require any special technical knowledge, depends to a great extent on common sense and a shrewd judgement of character, coupled with the capability of subverting fear."[108]

-Captain Alexander Stewart

Shortly after the beginning of World War I, a disturbing phenomenon began to appear. Young men from the front lines were being returned to field hospitals with strange symptoms that had never before been seen in war: Paralysis, in their legs, sometimes arms, without any observable wounds. An inability to speak. An inability to respond to verbal commands. Difficulty seeing. Sleeplessness. Anxiety.

These symptoms were attributed to the concussive effect of the explosions. Others speculated it was perhaps due to the toxic fumes which accompanied the fireball from the blast. At that time, unexplained illnesses would often be attributed to neurasthenia, and this would be no different. Doctors began associating the strange group of symptoms with the catch-all neurological diagnosis.

How might a soldier of this era have received any more medicinal metal than was typical of a civilian at that time? Besides smallpox, a Typhoid vaccine would likely have been the only immunizations a World War I soldier received,[i] shots not known for their mercury or aluminum content. But there was one source of metal most soldiers would have received—syphilis treatments.

The sexually transmitted infection was so prevalent and debilitating that during the 21 months the U.S. Army fought in World War I, it was estimated to have lost 6.8 million man days to its ill effects and treatment.[109] Until the 1940s, when penicillin was invented, the most popular treatments for syphilis were arsenic and mercury. These two metals would have been administered to anyone showing signs of a potential syphilis infection, and possibly even before.

Anyone alive in Europe or the United States during that time was likely to have had a fairly high baseline of metal toxicity entering the war. Add some very concerned military medical authorities to the mix and we can expect that many of these young men would have had stratospheric mercury and arsenic levels in their body.

Six months into World War I, 15% of British soldiers were thought to be unfit for service due to this neurasthenia-related problem. Nearly all of them had no medical explanation, other than their proximity to the explosions of artillery fire (both the firing of and the receiving of). As an initial report would observe, "Prolonged fatigue and exhaustion, coupled with continuous shelling, seem to be the primary causes of these mental breakdowns."[110] *Shell shock* became a catch-all term for the myriad of issues soldiers in the first World War were experiencing.

---

i. As of 1904, portions of the manufacture of anti-typhoid inoculation used mercury chloride as a disinfectant, but apparently lysol and carbonic acid were used as a preservative for multi-dose vials. It is conceivable they switched to mercury before World War I.

A 1917 film produced by British army neurologist Arthur Hurst[ii] called "War Neuroses" was one of the first times cinema had been used to document medical research and treatment techniques. Grainy clips of men with uncontrollable tremors, twitching faces and other neurological effects horrified those who saw them and erased any fantasies they may have had of the heroism of battle.

To the modern reader, it may seem like shell shock was one of the many inevitable horrors of war, but to the military leadership, the physicians attempting treatment, and even the civilians reading about it —it was clear this was something unique, something no one had ever seen before. It became such a public relations nightmare that later in World War II, the term was banned from being used within the military.

An army doctor named Charles Myers was tasked with treating these poor men and submitted a paper to The Lancet describing the details regarding three cases of shell shock.

Case 1
"Private, aged 20 … He was now retiring over open ground, kneeling on both knees and trying to creep under wire entanglements, when two or three shells burst near him. As he was struggling to disentangle himself from the wire three more shells burst behind and one in front of him. (An eye-witness in this hospital says that his escape was a sheer miracle.) After the shells had burst he succeeded in getting back under the wire entanglements ; all his comrades had retired already."

Case 2
"Corporal, aged 25. Admitted on Dec. 11th, 1914. The

---

ii. Arthur Hertz anglicized his name to Hurst after taking offense at the German aggressions of World War I.

*patient says that he was buried for 18 hours on Dec. 8th owing
to a shell bursting and "blowing in" the trench in which he lay.
Can remember nothing until he found himself in a dressing
station at a barn lying on straw."*

    Case 3
    *"Private, aged 23. Admitted on Jan. 26th, 1915. The patient
says that he was blown off a heap of bricks 15 feet high owing to
a shell bursting close to him. Thinks he must have fallen into a
pool of water, as he next remembers finding himself, about 3
P.M. the same afternoon, in a cellar near a church with his
clothes drenched."*[111]

By the end of the first world war, shell shock was a concept that,
due in large part to the "War Neuroses" film, was lodged in people's
minds as the inevitable result of suffering never-ending explosions of
war. But as the war progressed, new information surfaced that
confused those trying to understand the mechanisms of shell shock:
Many of the soldiers had never been within range of any artillery fire.
There had been no concussions, no gaseous fireballs. Not even machine
gun fire to have rattled their nerves, yet men were being carried in
ambulances to field hospitals with all of the mysterious symptoms. It
became clear that shell shock was not a physical injury, but a
neurological one.

War is stressful. As Lieutenant and Neurologist T. R. Elliot would
say in his early 1914 report:

    *"In some cases it is undoubtedly correct, for hysterical and
neurasthenic breakdowns are frequently met with in men who
have been exposed to the shattering effects of the great German
shells."*[112]

* * *

The effects of little to no sleep, constant physical exertion with poor nutrition would take its toll on the healthiest men our country could offer. But cannon fire was not a new military tactic in 1915 and had been used in battle for over 700 years. Something was different about this war and the men who fought it. An ominous difference which I believe would foretell the appearance of another unexplainable neurological illness—autism—many years later.

The first World War differed from most conflicts before and after not in technology or death toll, but in tactics. Earlier wars were fought in open fields of battle, where keeping one's distance might be considered the main defensive device. Later wars would rely on camouflage and subterfuge to provide cover.

World War I was fought chiefly from within trenches, long muddy ditches that snaked their way across Europe, often less than one hundred yards from their adversaries. Death was everywhere. Besides the constant threat of snipers, engineers might stealthily dig and place a collection of mines under a trench, blowing up the entire company. Airplanes flew overhead, logging their location for the artillery fire that would soon follow. Lice and rats shared the trenches with the soldiers and there was little they could do to keep them out. The stench of feces, urine and decaying bodies that littered the ground was pervasive. A single line from a soldier's diary summed it better than anyone could, "He who had a corpse to stand on was lucky."[113]

Rain worked against the soldiers as it turned the ground not into mud, but a thick sludge that could freeze at night and entrap the men for hours as they struggled to free themselves from the suction without alerting enemy snipers, ready to fire on anything showing signs of movement.

And there was nothing they could do about any of it. One soldier was a tiny cog in a great machine, and the only offense they could offer would be from charging over the top of their trench into a barrage of machine gun fire that would likely rip them to pieces. Running the other way, even in cowardly retreat, would likely suffer them the same fate. Yet those maddening options of escape, through victory or death, were denied to them. Weeks could pass without a significant change in strategy. They were to stay where they were and wait for further instructions—instructions that might come a day later, or a month later, once half of their fellow soldiers had already died from sniper fire, dysentery, or suicide.

Research into the factors that cause stress have grouped them into three common categories: uncertainty, the lack of information and the loss of control.[114] Besides the constant threat of death itself, trench warfare in this era would seem to be capable of creating all of these perfectly. Additionally, the weeks and months-long engagement of their primal fight or flight response would have created chronic immune activation in portions of their brain. But there was something about World War 1 and these cases of shell shock that felt more than a just a simple prolonged fight or flight response.

AUTISM & BABIES

The onset of autism is frequently associated with young children, particularly between the ages of thirteen and eighteen months. An older child or adult may occasionally develop some sort of neurological disorder, but autism nearly always appears in babies. If autism is not from a virus or bacteria taking advantage of the weak immune response of an infant, why might it happen so often at this particular age? The stories of shell-shock from World War I would begin to form a very clear picture of why this happens.

Fight or flight is a natural response to the threat of injury. The human brain, like other animals, signals the appropriate autonomic and immunologic response to this perceived danger. The response is to fight or to flee. One or the other. But the soldiers of World War I, stuck for weeks, sometimes months, under horrifying conditions of the trenches, both inside and out, had an additional survival instinct that was being triggered, something that had never happened before.

The oppressive sensation of being stuck is unmistakable from reading accounts of the horrors these young men suffered through.

Think back to the three original accounts mentioned in the previous chapter: Case 1) Tangled in barbed wire as shells exploded nearby. 2) Half-buried within his collapsed trench for 18 hours as shells burst around him. 3) Thrown from a pile of bricks into a pool of water with no memory of what happened, ostensibly knocked senseless while fighting to get out of the water.

As you read through many of the cases of what was called shell shock at that time, you cannot help but notice a recurring theme: Trapped, with no chance of escape. You cannot stand up, you cannot move. You cannot go forward, you cannot go backward. Death will find you if you try. Death will find you if you don't. The psychological toll of weeks of this madness cannot be overestimated.

As it turns out, recent psychological research into this phenomenon would offer a third and final reason the dorsal vagal complex was being triggered—something that would keep me awake for days.

Remember that I had been searching for a reason why the dorsal vagal complex was being immune activated. The dorsal vagal complex is that special location in the brain stem where many of the body's most important cranial nerves emanate from. Recently injected aluminum from vaccines moves around the body inside white blood cells via the blood and lymphatic system. Directly after injections, there is a higher amount of these aluminum-containing white blood cells because many of them have not yet found a resting place inside muscle tissue or been encapsulated inside granulomas.

I believe the reason acute cranial nerve damage is so common after vaccination is because the aluminum is free to travel to the dorsal vagal complex—as long as the body's immune system *signals* for it to go there. As I searched for answers as to why the immune system might signal for help at the dorsal vagal complex, I found two answers right away: pathogen invasion and tissue injury. Those two events—which happen anytime a child is vaccinated— would trigger immune activation within the dorsal vagal complex and cause a signal to go out to the body for help from white blood cells—many of which that would unfortunately contain aluminum.

Pathogen invasion and tissue injury alone would be enough reason we see so many acute neurological issues after metals are injected into the body. But they don't explain why babies or toddlers seem so susceptible to assault. Many adults get vaccines and there is usually little neurological risk—you rarely see an adult experiencing anything like autism after their shots. Why is it that the younger children seem more vulnerable to cranial nerve damage after vaccination? Why would their dorsal vagal complex signal for help so aggressively?

As it turns out, the fight or flight mechanism is only the first step in the body's response to danger. There are situations in which neither fight *nor* flight are possible options, and in these rare cases, an older, more primal sequence of events happens.

I first heard about Polyvagal theory from a gastroenterologist who had spent a good bit of his retirement researching the causes of autism. As I was sharing some of my early theories with him, he dug up a paper that he and another scientist had collaborated on. It discussed the possibility of autism originating in the brainstem,[115] and a portion of polyvagal theory factors heavily into their paper.

Proposed by Dr. Stephen Porges, polyvagal theory attempts to understand the nature of the sympathetic and para-sympathetic nervous systems in our body and how they relate to stress responses. When the initial fight or flight reaction fails to produce a satisfactory stress response, the body transitions into another phase.

According to Dr. Porges, this second phase, referred to as *death feigning*, occurs as "… an adaptive response to life threat when options for fight/ flight behaviors are minimized, such as during restraint or when there is an inability to escape."[116] This behavior is exhibited by possums when they "play dead" and is not voluntary—they are not pretending to be dead—their body has actually created a massive set of dorsal vagal instructions that can slow the heart rate down, trigger paralysis, or even spontaneous defecation in some animals.

This response which originates in the dorsal vagal complex is a primitive, last-ditch effort to save the animals life when it has become obvious that fight or flight do not present meaningful options for survival.

As I began to comprehend the implications of this survival mechanism, the World War I soldiers and the symptoms of their suffering suddenly made sense to me. Initially, they had attributed their strange new symptoms to the effects of concussions from the explosions of the artillery shells. But as the war dragged on, it became apparent many of the soldiers suffering from shell shock had never been fired on with artillery shells at all.

These young men *had* been put in a situation where fight or flight was impossible. They could neither advance, nor retreat. They had been perpetually stuck in fight or flight mode for weeks, months at a time, with no option for escape. Even the barbed wire and mud created further restraint.

For those who did experience the trauma of having a shell explode right next to them, many of them went into a primal freeze described exactly by polyvagal theory. Their legs, sometimes their arms, would appear to be completely paralyzed. Their hearing, their vision—gone. They were catatonic—completely unable to move or speak for hours, sometimes more. Eventually, after resting for a few days, their movement would return, their ability to hear and speak apparently restored.

But the other symptoms which didn't go away—symptoms that men who had never even seen a shell explode experienced—could probably be attributed to a more unfortunate circumstance. The immune activation—created in their dorsal vagal complex by the tissue injury of war and their months-long inability to escape from a perceived threat from life in the trenches—acted like a beacon, signaling any available metals they had in their body to their brain.

As the horror of how this primal response to threat might inadvertently be summoning metal directly to the brain became obvious, another realization struck me. There were others. It wasn't just the World War I soldiers. There were others who were being put in fight or flight mode and given no option for escape. But unlike the soldiers, they were being given a massive amount of metal at the exact same time as their dorsal vagal activation.

IMMOBILIZATION. RESTRAINT.

I had just shared the concept of immobilization and restraint as a trigger for activating the dorsal vagal complex in a video online, and a few people wrote me with some of their stories.

"My daughter was getting her four year old shots... The nurse held her down and stuck her with the first shot and she screamed and threw herself away from the nurse and she had to get 3 other nurses to hold her arms and legs down. She tried to get me to hold her but I couldn't and would not! It was awful! She screamed so loud everyone in the whole office and waiting room could hear her. She kept begging me to make it stop but I didn't know what to do. That stupid nurse stabbed her repeatedly with the needle because she kept jumping. I saw the fluid ooze back out of the needle holes because she was struggling so bad. I was crying, My daughter was screaming and my husband didn't know what to do either! I said enough at the fifth shot but she stabbed my daughter with the sixth anyways!

We were all crying as we went out to the car. We sat there in complete shock! It was so horrible, traumatic. I hate to compare it to rape but the violence that took place left us scarred for life. I had nightmares for years after, my daughter too and my husband said never again. My daughter couldn't walk for three days. Her legs were swollen from her hips down to her ankles. Her fever was 104.2. I thought we would have to take her to the hospital but we didn't."

Many older people have clear memories of getting shots at school. I remember being in first grade and seeing kids from another class lining up to get a shot outside. When I got home I was terrified and told my mom what was happening. She told me that I was going to have to get a shot the next day, and I cried for hours—I was absolutely terrified. I was seven years old and was struggling to come up with something—anything I could think of to get out of the shot.

The next day, I could think about nothing else and felt like my heart was going to explode out of my chest. We were led out of the classroom and lined up outside in the courtyard. I could see the nurse walking down the line towards me, motioning for everyone to roll their sleeves up.

"I don't want the shot," I whispered to her as she approached, my eyes tearing up. "I don't want it."

"It'll be okay," she said. "You'll barely feel it."

I had not thought of that day for a very long time until I watched the film "Schindler's List." There was a scene where men, women and children had just gotten off the train and were being lined up and asked questions about their skills and abilities, a question which—although they didn't know it—would determine if they would live or die. Somehow, the panic and anxiety they must have felt resonated with me because of that shot day at school many years ago.

Another woman wrote with her account of a school-administered vaccine.

"I can remember another time when myself and the rest of the class were vaccinated at my elementary school in CA in the nurse's office. I remember everyone lining up and then everyone crying their eyes out in the halls afterwards. This was about 3rd grade for me. It was one shot and it's not on my record. Days later I had the highest fever my body and my brain had ever had at 106.3 and I started hallucinating and fading in and out of consciousness. I remember shaking violently and falling in and out... I had a weird form of anxiety develop after this vaccine, where one of the chambers of my heart would pain if I take a deep breath. I also suffer from auditory hallucinations still to this day (I'm 26 now), where I can hear the hallucination I had from that vaccine when I'm stressed or nervous."

The long-term effects of some of these shot visits are obvious from reading accounts like this:

"Whenever people crowd around me, say in an elevator or small room, or are in my personal bubble, I can feel those nurses hands on me again, and the way the exam table was cold and I hear the paper rustle in my ears, and smell the overpowering odor of iodine/rubbing alcohol. It just makes me feel physically ill. The few times I've taken my own children into a clinic for various things, I have to focus on a spot on the wall or else I get sucked into a terrible walk down memory lane."

The details—smells or sounds, they all can trigger these horrible memories. One women shared the story of her natural instincts to protect being violated by an uncaring nurse:

✳ ✳ ✳

"I decided it might help to keep her close to me, to hold her if possible, when she had to be treated or examined or get tested or shots. I would kiss her cheek, whisper in her ears, sing, and gently stoke her hair or cheek or arm, back, or leg to comfort and distract her. Until she was about 1-year-old and a nurse grabbed her from me and insisted I could not hold her as she took her away from me and abruptly put her on a cold table... I was devastated to see my child crying sooo hard... In that thoughtless, uncaring moment that woman changed both our lives! I will not forget her or forgive her for the manner of disregard and disrespect in which she handled that situation by not allowing me to nurture my child thru a process most children and even adults will report as distasteful and uncomfortable and worse."

These are just a few of the stories people shared with me. For many parents, whose children were injured because of this process, it is too painful to think about. Regardless, this is why I propose that babies suffer neurologic injury after vaccines much more often than adults— or even older kids, for that matter. Humans have a primal instinct against being stabbed—no surprise there—and little children have no idea you are trying to help them, despite your reassuring smiles and lollipops or milkshakes. Even once they're older it can be difficult, but for a young child who doesn't understand what's going on, they are going to be very afraid.

A child will certainly cycle through the fight or flight stress response and the parent or nurse's restraint may send them into the next—something which will activate their dorsal vagal complex. This will happen to some extent whether the restraint is required or not, simply due to the other two triggers happening—pathogen invasion and tissue injury. If you add the third one due to immobilization and restraint, you will end up with a massively activated dorsal vagal complex.

Most adults will not activate the third trigger and as a result will not receive the massive amount of white blood cells to their brainstem as a child might. This is not true for everyone, as a few children seem to have an extremely high pain tolerance and can be easily distracted. Similarly, a few adults have an understandable fear of needles that may never go away.

Shots obviously hurt, but the psychological effects of your parents pinning you down so that you can be stabbed is traumatic—much more traumatic than people realize. No one enjoys this process—doctors, nurses, parents or children, but it was always assumed that "the end justifies the means." The mechanisms described in polyvagal theory, and their potential impact on the safety of injecting metals into children's bodies may force us to reconsider that statement.

You may insist on vaccinating your children, even after considering the dangers of injected metal presented in this book. If you are this person, I would ask you to please consider learning to recognize the signs of infection early, learn some healthy alternatives to vaccination, but most importantly wait to vaccinate your children until they are old enough to understand.

If your children require restraint in order to administer shots, then in my opinion, they are too young to be safely immunized. This restraint will trigger their dorsal vagal complex in such a way as to signal the metals that were just injected into their bodies straight to vulnerable parts of their brain. Wait until they are old enough to understand, then make a decision with them regarding vaccines.

WHY DON'T GIRLS GET AUTISM?

Just after World War II had ended, a medical researcher from Cambridge University named Elsie Widdowson was working in Germany to monitor the health and nutrition of children who had lost their parents in the war. The children's fare had improved, but years of living on meager rations had taken their toll, and many of the children were severely underweight.

Sensing an opportunity for scientific study, Elsie and her colleagues wanted to see how much a slight improvement in the children's rations would affect their ability to thrive. There were two orphanages, each with about fifty children in them. One of the orphanages was given extra orange juice, bread and jelly. After six months, their heights and weights were measured and their gains compared with the other orphanage.

Incredibly, the orphanage with the regular rations showed the most gains. They had less food but had clearly grown more. The orphanage where the kids had been given more food showed very little gains. Confused, and perhaps feeling a little guilty, the researchers switched the rations for another six months and then measured again.

Just like before, the results were the opposite of what they would have expected. The original orphanage, now getting less food rather than more, was showing more growth, while the other orphanage on extra rations had stalled. The researchers—many of whom had done careful study of nutrition—were completely stumped. What could explain why less food was causing more growth in both sets of children?

As it would turn out, it had nothing to do with the food, but with the two Frauleins who were in charge of the orphanages. By coincidence, somewhere near the end of the first six months, one of them was promoted to the more prominent orphanage due to the constant care and compassion she showed to the children. The woman she replaced, known for her steely temper and the fear she could create in her charges, was demoted—to the other orphanage.

In other words, they switched places—at about the exact time the rations were changed. Fraulein Grun had twice overseen fifty orphans with less food and the nurture she provided them showed up in scientific data that couldn't be explained any other way. Similarly, the fear and stress the other Fraulein meted out stunted the children's growth and probably negatively affected their health in other ways.

These results initially stunned researchers, because they had been taught that food and exercise are what cause human growth. Incredibly, a woman's tending instinct appeared to be as important to the children's growth as food. It occurred that nurturing shouldn't just be considered a nicety that a few lucky children received, but an essential component of a healthy upbringing—not just some pie-in-the-sky notion of mental health, but actual physical wellbeing.

With these facts in mind, scientists have begun to look anew at *motherhood* less with a nostalgic, misty-eyed homage and more with an attempt at an empirical understanding of the hormones and other biological processes at play. A study looking at the effects of hypertension—something that's considered a genetic trait—also revealed something surprising about nurturing.[117] A group of young rat pups who were bred to develop hypertension were split in half. One group was nursed by mothers who also had been bred to develop hypertension, while the other group was given to mothers who were not. Once they matured, testing revealed the hypertensive pups who had been given to the "normal" mothers showed no signs of hypertension while the other group did. As Shelley Taylor says in her book, *The Tending Instinct*, "A mother's tending can completely eliminate the expression of a genetic heritage."[118]

Taylor and her colleagues made an interesting observation as she tried to reckon her own personal experiences with what the scientific literature was saying about human behavior, particularly the response to stress. Whether it was due to chauvinism or out of genuine concern, most psychological studies that had been done did not include female subjects. "The sudden recognition that all of the classic theories of stress were based almost entirely on males was a stunning revelation."[119]

Ashley Smith was opening her apartment door late one night in 2005 when a man with a gun pushed her inside and locked the door behind them. Ashley recognized him from television newscasts—he was Brian Nichols and had escaped from a courthouse by overpowering a guard and grabbing his gun. He had already shot and killed a judge, a deputy sheriff, a journalist and a federal agent who was chasing him. Ashely would make five.

She was tied up in the bathroom and couldn't move. She thought of her daughter, 5, who could become an orphan as her husband had been killed several years earlier. During the night, she convinced her captor to allow her to read a book to him—*The Purpose Driven Life*. She was able to connect with him through some of the passages in the book that spoke to pain they had both suffered.

By the morning, Ashley had earned enough trust from Nichols that he allowed her to go pick up her daughter. Once safely in the car, she called 911 and Nichols was apprehended.

Over the past twenty or thirty years, additional behavioral studies have been conducted and this time they included females. Some of the results revealed that women can sometimes have a very different response to stress than men. Whereas the default behavior for men is the Fight or Flight response—evidenced by an increased heart rate, increased respiration, the dilation of eyes and others—women exhibit a different sequence of hormonal and biological events. Probably not surprising to women reading this, but science can sometimes take a while to catch up.

> ”*The dominant metaphor, 'fight or flight,' represents the threatening social landscape as a solitary kill-or-be-killed world. My work suggests instead that the human response to stress is characterized at least as much by tending to and befriending others, a pattern that is especially true of women.*”[120]

Put another way, women under stress are more likely to turn to friends, family, loved ones, even strangers, for help. Rather than going into fight or flight, females are inclined towards what is sometimes called "tend and befriend." You can imagine that with a child at your side and an infant at your breast, fighting or fleeing do not present very good options for any of your children's survival. Threatening situations actually evoke tending behaviors, even to the point where women can develop strong bonds with complete strangers that might otherwise harm them.

Oxytocin, sometimes called the cuddle hormone, is not only used to initiate labor and milk production, but is also released in times of stress. Researchers injected female sheep with oxytocin and tracked their maternal behaviors, such as touching and grooming. All of them increased after the injections.[121]

If someone were to generate a massive amount of oxytocin during a stressful event, it might explain why some women's tending instincts overtake their desire to fight or flee. With additional stress, other hormones can flood the body. *Endogenous Opioid Peptides* (EOPs) are associated with the euphoric "runner's high" and the suppression of pain. Social contact, even physical touching, can generate these EOPs and lessen the sensation of physical pain.

Females behave differently than males under stress. It doesn't mean their heart rates do not go up and it doesn't mean they do not experience the fight or flight sensation or freezing. But according to *The Tending Instinct* author, who went through 30 different studies looking at the difference between male and female responses to stress:

> "*The difference between women's and men's inclination to turn to the social group in times of stress ranks with 'giving birth' as among the most reliable sex differences there are.*"[122]

I believe these extreme differences in response to stress are the main reason that girls develop autism and other neurological disorders four times less frequently than boys. Recall that I am proposing the majority of acute damage associated with autism originates in the dorsal vagal complex. It may spread outward from that area into other cranial nerves, but that is where it begins. Why? Because the stress from being pinned down and being injected with a pathogen cause precisely the three things known to trigger the dorsal vagal complex: pathogen invasion, tissue injury, and restraint or immobilization.

When the dorsal vagal complex is immune activated, it signals for help which the body supplies via white blood cells—except in the age of medicine and metals, our white blood cells carry aluminum inside. The white blood cells will penetrate the dorsal vagal complex where they may die a natural death, exposing the aluminum inside to the cranial nerve nuclei, causing damage in the form of lesions to the nerve tissue.

According to my theory, the hormonal changes females experience under stress is what saves them from the neurological injury males so often experience. The dorsal vagal complex is not activated in girls the same way it is with boys. Girls, upon threat of harm may go into "tend and befriend" mode which has a different sequence of immunological events associated with it, such as the release of Oxytocin. If the threat increases, females may begin to release EOPs, the hormone designed to alleviate pain and increase bonding.

Because a female's dorsal vagal complex is not immune activated the way it is in males during stress, it does not signal aggressively for help, thus saving them from the brunt of an aluminum assault. Pathogen invasion and tissue injury will trigger their dorsal vagal complex—there is apparently little difference in gender between those first two triggers. But the third—immobilization and restraint—is apparently a very strong trigger in males.

Tending and befriending sounds like a horrible response to stress on the surface, but when you think of it in terms of saving and preserving children, it sounds like a perfect biochemical explanation for the care and sacrifice that mothers are famous for. The reason that girls typically don't develop autism or other neurological injuries from vaccines is a beautiful testament to their tending, nurturing design. And as beautiful as that explanation may be, it's equally horrible when you realize the opposite response that 2 or 4 or 12 or 18-month-old boys have is also designed to save, protect and preserve their future children. But their reaction to immobilization and restraint—unlike the female's tend and befriend response—is what sends out a signal for help, a signal that aluminum-containing white blood cells are all too happy to answer.

This is why girls don't get much neurological injury from the aluminum in vaccines. This is also why you don't see many girls with crooked faces. The lopsided smile and the misaligned eyes are much more common in boys, just like autism. The crooked face is an early warning sign of neurological injury—it will often show up before anything else does. Not always, but often.

Young girls receive the same amount of injected aluminum that boys do, but it often gets safely stored away inside granulomas. These granulomas cannot protect forever, and often begin to fail during their teenage years, when autoimmune diseases so often appear. Before we discuss the nature of many of these disorders that so often affect females, I need to highlight one last obvious source of male-specific dorsal vagal complex activation.

THE CIRCUMSTRAINT

Many of you probably immediately thought of the effects of circumcision on an infant boy. Without delving into a debate on the merits of the *outcome* of the operation, the procedure itself offers plenty of opportunity for concern.

The same three triggers for activating the dorsal vagal complex we see during vaccination are present: pathogen invasion, tissue injury and restraint. The tissue injury associated with circumcision is probably obvious but the other two may not be. Local anesthetics are injected into the boy's genitals to numb them for the operation. While these anesthetics have the effect of lessening the pain associated with the procedure, the body will see them as pathogens—foreign invaders—and will trigger the dorsal vagal complex in response. Lastly, the boys are strapped into a restraining device that completely immobilizes them so that the procedure can be done safely.

For most, this procedure is done before their son leaves the hospital —a seemingly trivial event among many others which boys must go through before they are released. During my research on the activation of the dorsal vagal complex, images of the Circumstraint—a popular product for restraining baby boys during circumcision—haunted me. It was light brown plastic, a vague anthropomorphic form that a baby could be strapped into, their legs held slightly apart. If the device were made of wood and its sterile, medical aesthetic removed—it would be a fitting prop from a terrifying horror movie.

The only thing that gave me comfort was the thought that infant babies were so young and immobile that the restraint was unnecessary. Perhaps it was only for "just in case" they made a sudden movement from pain. I began to see pictures that wrecked me—infant boys with their eyes glassed over. They were not under general anesthesia—they were fully awake, but frozen. Catatonic. The restraint *was* necessary. They had cycled through fight or flight, if only with the most miniscule, weak effort they could summon, and had apparently transitioned into death feigning—the same primal response to restraint and immobilization that animals, reptiles and even World War I soldiers exhibit.

This act may seem barbaric as stated, but in light of another event may cross the line into the diabolical. If the boy was born in the United States, just hours, if not minutes before this procedure is done, he is likely to have received a hepatitis B vaccine—even though it's a disease typically transmitted by sexual contact or sharing needles. This vaccine contains a significant amount of aluminum, the neurotoxin—enough to kill if it were delivered to the right spot in the brain. Luckily, it rarely does.

After the shot is administered, it is followed up with another dorsal vagal complex trigger—circumcision. These two assaults on the brains (and bodies) of infant boys, not even hours old, disturb me. Without the pale green scrubs, linoleum floors and fluorescent lights, circumcision might appear to be the rites of a satanic ritual.

Regardless of the outcome of this surgery, the way the procedure is performed and the timing of it all cannot be sustained by a civilized society for long. As I mentioned in another chapter about restraining children for vaccines, if I were to have a baby boy, I would let them decide on the procedure themselves. Let them grow up and make an informed decision about their own body when they are old enough to understand the consequences and not require restraint during the procedure.

DISEASES OF METAL & MICROBES

"I had been my whole life a bell, and never knew it until at that moment I was lifted and struck."

— *Annie Dillard, Pilgrim at Tinker Creek*

The disorders listed in this section may form in the presence of metal, microbes, and in some cases, antibiotics. You will notice many of these diseases are not purely neurological but are more systemic, affecting everything including joints, skin, intestines, lungs, and other organs. Where acute metal toxicity seems to occur in very specific areas of the brain, the combination of metals and microbes create long-running infections that allow the symptoms of chronic inflammation to move around the body.

ALLERGIES & ASTHMA

*"We are in need of a new, general, nonprejudicial word to
designate the altered condition which an organism achieves after
acquaintance with an organic, living, or inanimate poison."*

- Clemens von Pirquet, 1906

Allergies and asthma are such a common ailment that modern humans are likely to think they have always existed, alongside smallpox or the common cold. "The rates may be increasing," they might admit, but allergy or asthma in one form or another has been a constant source of irritation—indeed a deadly threat to others—for all of human history.

It turns out like crooked faces, allergies and asthma are a relatively recent phenomenon. In 1819, around the same time Charles Bell was beginning to understand the nerve palsies that had been affecting people's faces, another doctor in London announced some peculiar new symptoms he had personally experienced:

> *"About the beginning or middle of June in every year the following symptoms make their appearance, with a greater or less degree of violence... A sensation of heat and fulness is experienced in the eyes... a general fulness is experienced in the head, and particularly about 'the forepart; to this succeeds irritation of the nose, producing sneezing'... To the sneezings are added a farther sensation of tightness of the chest, and a difficulty of breathing..."*[123]

You may instantly recognize this particular suffering as "seasonal allergies," something that used to be called *hay fever*, but this doctor and all of those listening to his presentation didn't recognize it—none of them had ever heard of anything like it before. Even ten years later, when he presented again to the same group, he still had found no mention of this very peculiar illness in the medical literature despite an exhaustive search. None of the "most eminent" physicians he met with in London, Liverpool or Edinburgh had heard of it—it was as if hay fever had appeared out of thin air:

> *"One of the most remarkable circumstances respecting this complaint is its not having been noticed as a specific affection, until within the last ten or twelve years. Except a single observation of Heberden's*, I have not met with anything that can be supposed to refer to it in any author, ancient or modern."*[124]

By the second presentation in 1828, he *had* been able to find 28 local cases and provided some of the details of their suffering. In an account that would later mirror cases of *infantile paralysis*[i], the

---

i. Later called polio.

affliction seemed to target the more affluent ranks of society:

> "It is remarkable, that all the cases are in the middle or
> upper classes of society, some indeed of high rank. I have made
> inquiry at the various dispensaries in London and elsewhere,
> and I have not heard of a single unequivocal case occurring
> among the poor."[125]

It was clear that hay fever was a new illness. It was also clear its rates were increasing. And like the many other diseases that began to appear during the early 1800s, no one could explain why they were happening nor seemed to have treatments that could help.

Over time, hay fever has become synonymous with *allergic rhinitis*, an umbrella diagnosis for the many different seasonal allergies people suffer from these days. Eventually, scientists were able to figure out that pollen—not hay—was the provocateur. Other triggers would later be discovered such as mold, dust and pet hair, but like *hay-asthma*, hay-fever was unheard of until the early 1800s.

In fact, the terms allergy or anaphylaxis didn't exist within our language at that time. A few references appear to mention unnaturally strong reactions to an insect sting, but that was it. Besides hay fever, the concept of allergy would remain completely foreign to medical literature until the very late 1800s.

In what must have seemed an unremarkable coincidence, there was a new medical treatment—invented 20 years earlier and just miles away —that had begun to gain popularity. It was called *vaccination*, and by scraping the scabs or pus from a farm animal (usually a cow) sick with *cowpox* into your arm, it was supposed to allow you to safely generate immunity to a much deadlier version of the disease—*smallpox*.

This concept was initially met with horror by many. The poor could not afford it, but those who could were already reluctant to let a mercury-happy doctor treat them. At the time, any new medical treatment that didn't kill you or cause your teeth to fall out might be considered a technological marvel. Although the vaccine had its share of nasty side effects—like full-body eczema (another world first)—it was deemed safe enough and gained larger acceptance by the end of the 1800s as more people began to allow doctors to cut their arm and rub the "ingredients" into the wound.[ii]

Clues as to how the smallpox vaccine might be causing hay fever would not emerge for almost another hundred years. In the 1890s scientists began work on developing a *diphtheria* antitoxin—what is now the "D" in DTaP and TDaP shots. Similar to the techniques they were using to create tetanus antitoxin, they would inject a horse with increasing doses of the diphtheria toxin until it had developed antibodies in its blood. They would bleed the horse, filter out the red blood cells and take the remaining liquid—optimistically referred to as "serum"—and inject it into children in hopes of protecting them from diphtheria.

There was a danger with this process—the horse blood contained a million other things in it—things which our immune system would never encounter naturally. The first response to having this diphtheria antitoxin, or horse blood serum, injected into a child's body could sometimes create a mild response. But the second one could sometimes create a massive, life threatening reaction.

They didn't know it at the time, but the first injection had resulted in minor side effects as the immune system created antibodies to the foreign material. When injected a second time, the immune system now recognized the invader and created a response so violent it could kill. During their attempt to understand what was causing it, French and German scientists coined two terms to describe these new

---

ii. Another technique was to "sew" a needle and pus-soaked thread through the skin of an arm. Interestingly, doctors would mail smallpox scabs to each other for generating vaccines.

phenomena – *allergy* and *anaphylaxis*.[iii] These horrible reactions were a common effect of the diphtheria antitoxin—over 40% of injections created this allergy response, according to public health officials at the time.[126]

The world now had perhaps two allergies, both of them due to injections—the hay fever of smallpox, and the allergic response to materials in the diphtheria shot. Like bee stings and snake bites, injections allow foreign material to bypass your body's main defense system—the mucosal tissue—where they can invoke an allergic response with ease. Some vaccines are still developed using animals such as the flu shot, often grown in racks of chicken eggs. Drug manufacturers have become more skilled at filtering out unwanted material, but allergies can easily be created with many different materials simply by injecting them into your bloodstream.

Modern filtration has minimized the chance of creating allergy from the ingredients in vaccination, but other ingredients can inadvertently maximize a reaction to any allergen by a chance exposure. This created a very big problem, as could be seen in the explosion of food allergies that began to appear in the 1930s.[127]

Aluminum, the adjuvant used in vaccines, works well specifically because your body reacts so strongly to it. It's often used in scientific experiments because it amplifies the immune response to allergens.[128] In a 2007 experiment, researchers were able to create an allergy in mice simply by injecting them with a codfish extract alongside a common aluminum-containing antacid.[129] For years, researchers have been able to induce asthma in mice by injecting *ovalbumin*[iv] alongside aluminum hydroxide.[130] They've also been able to create dust mite-induced asthma using the same method,[131] and exposure to aluminum has even been

iii. Scientists even coined a slang term for it: Serum sickness.
iv. Egg white protein.

238

shown to cause asthma in humans.[132]

Whether it's food exposure in your gut, or aerosolized exposure in your lungs and sinuses, the modern age of medicine seems at least capable of creating the hundreds of different allergies that have appeared in the last eighty years.

It is impossible to speak of allergies and not mention the peanut, the cause of so much suffering amongst children of today. For someone who has developed an allergy to peanuts, exposure can be life threatening. If you've never witnessed a child gasping desperately for air from exposure to a tiny amount of this seemingly benign legume, it's difficult to understand the fear both child and parent must live with every day.

Peanut allergy is a modern problem that doesn't appear to have existed in any medical literature until the late 1940s. A 1941 book on food allergy titled "Strange Malady" attempted to explain what it called "this strange illness."[133] A partial list of problematic foods the author identified were milk, egg, corn, soybean, cottonseed, shrimp, tomato, cabbage, cherry, chocolate, and strawberries. Peanut allergies were notably absent, but would soon make an appearance just a few years later in 1950 after a study on injected penicillin revealed that an ingredient used in the manufacture of the new antibiotic—peanut oil—was causing peanut allergies for children in the test.[134][v]

For many, the milk, egg or shrimp allergies they had begun to experience were an annoyance. Peanuts were different. Their ability to harm appeared to be uniquely powerful as researchers have confirmed:

> *"Our observations, when combined with those published by other investigators, suggest that the high incidence, persistence*

---

v. Heather Fraser's "The Peanut Allergy Epidemic" is an excellent read on this topic.

and severity of peanut allergy may result from a combination of properties that make it a 'perfect' allergen..."[135]

Much speculation has been made over the contents of various pharmaceutical products over the years, as peanut oil was a frequent ingredient. There are so many stages to the manufacture of any modern drug or vaccine that it would be difficult to guarantee it to be absolutely free of any trace of peanut.

Maybe the bacteria-altering properties of certain antibiotics many kids are likely to receive today can create so many problems in their gut that food particles make it into their bloodstream. This may be why we sometimes see food allergy in unvaccinated children.

Perhaps it does not matter. Before the age of aluminum, peanuts may have been uniquely *unable* to create allergy without being injected, and even that direct assault created only a minor sensitivity compared with what we see in children of today. On the other hand, with a gut flush with aluminum, the allergenicity of peanuts—even by simple ingestion—might be catapulted into the vaunted status it occupies today.

Was the smallpox vaccine the cause of hay fever? As the ingredients of the vaccine are poorly understood, even today,[136] it is impossible to say, but given the remarkably similar timing and location of the appearance of this new illness (early 1800s London), it would appear likely. As the vaccine was discontinued in the 1970s,[vi] one might expect that the rates of hay fever should be going down, and in fact they appear to be doing just that. If you look up allergy statistics, you will discover that the age group of 18-44 year olds has slightly more than

---

vi. The smallpox vaccine was pulled in the 1970s not because the disease was declared eradicated but because the vaccine had so many horrible side effects.

half as much hay fever[vii] as the older groups[137]—people who would have received the smallpox vaccine.

I believe the smallpox vaccine, because it was grown in various animals, contained a unique component that created a pollen allergy in many of those who got the vaccine. This allergy would stand alone for a long time, an illness so unique that a more broad term—"allergy"— wasn't coined until 1904, nearly 85 years later.

In the 1900s, when aluminum began to be injected, its unique properties, though not understood, became apparent as people could develop allergies and asthmatic responses to nearly anything. As it turns out, asthma and allergies may be just two of the symptoms of a dysfunctional immune system caused by aluminum's ability to modify the body's response to invaders. This realization would put a very unlikely set of diseases on the list beside asthma and allergies—Crohn's disease and ulcerative colitis.

---

vii. Survey respondents were asked by phone if they had been diagnosed with "hay fever." A true result that wasn't inadvertently representing the broader "seasonal allergies" category might be even smaller.

CROHN'S & ULCERATIVE COLITIS

If you or someone you know has not dealt with an *inflammatory bowel disease,* you may think of it as just another one of many annoyances of life—like a cold or the occasional flu. *Crohn's disease* and *ulcerative colitis* are debilitating diseases that can sometimes kill. For the two million Americans that suffer from these conditions, much of their day can be spent managing pain, malnutrition, and many other symptoms associated with badly dysfunctional guts.

Crohn's disease usually starts as inflammation at the *terminal ileum,* the point at which the small intestine connects to the large. It can spread from there—sometimes skipping areas—and in rare cases the disease can extend anywhere throughout the digestive tract. The inflammation from Crohn's can be fierce, pushing through the wall of the intestines, creating connections between organs that are not supposed to exist. Sometimes damaged portions of the intestines have to be removed, creating another set of problems the patient has to manage. Ulcerative colitis—or colitis—while usually less damaging than Crohn's, can still be a horrible illness to cope with. It is limited to the large intestine and usually occurs in a continuous pattern.

The description of what causes Crohn's disease as described by one of the leading charities for this illness will be familiar to nearly anyone who has suffered from autoimmune disorders:

> *"The causes of Crohn's disease are not well understood. Diet and stress may aggravate Crohn's Disease, but they do not cause the disease on their own. Recent research suggests hereditary, genetics, and/or environmental factors contribute to the development of Crohn's Disease."*[138]

Like many other disorders, the search for a genetic key that might unlock the door to a cure for Crohn's and ulcerative colitis has been frustrating. Anytime someone has a severely debilitating illness and their identical twin does not, you begin to suspect an environmental factor plays a more important role than genetics.

Inflammatory bowel diseases often have an onset that can be traced to a particular event: the stress of starting college, a bad infection, training for a marathon. The illness can flare up and cause all kinds of problems for months while those who are suffering try various dietary changes, antibiotics, steroids and biologics.

Sometimes they seem to work and the symptoms of the disease will lift—for months, sometimes years, only to come raging back into someone's life. Often when this happens, a new set of symptoms appears alongside—they may not be the same as last time, and the same treatments that worked before, now seem to do nothing. As it turns out, Crohn's and ulcerative colitis perfectly illustrate the damage that metals, microbes and medicine can wreak in someone's life.

It has been clear to researchers there is some type of microbial component to Crohn's. As far back as 1992, bacterial cultures were taken from those suffering from Crohn's inflammation and a common culprit was discovered: *Mycobacterium avium paratuberculosis*[139]—also called "Myco" or MAP.[i] In another study, MAP bacteria were injected into rabbits who developed inflammation in their ileum—the same spot where Crohn's often starts in humans. Researchers thought they had isolated the bacteria that was causing Crohn's disease. But there was a problem—Myco infections weren't consistent. They didn't always cause inflammation. People who previously had Crohn's disease could have active Myco bacteria in their blood but show few signs of active inflammation in their gut. Scientists were understandably confused and Myco bacteria, which had shown much promise in revealing the pathology of Crohn's, faded into the background while other research continued to look for genetic markers of the disease.

Another obscure study revealed a crucial clue to understanding not only Crohn's and ulcerative colitis, but nearly all of the chronic inflammation disorders listed in this book. The bacteria *Streptococcus faecalis* was placed into rabbit ileum but it failed to develop any of the symptoms of Crohn's. Then, the experiment was repeated, but with a cell wall deficient version of the *same* bacteria—the intracellular form. This time, the results were unmistakable—inflammation, just like with Crohn's.[140]

Bacteria in their natural state were unable to create Crohn's disease. But the same bacteria were able to cause inflammation if they existed in their intracellular state—the version *without* the cell wall. This was a huge clue that—similar to the discovery of Myco bacteria—held promise. Perhaps the problem was Myco bacteria could cause Crohn's inflammation, but only in their intracellular state. Research on this line of thinking stalled because again, the variables that seemed to trigger Crohn's disease were elusive. What was causing Myco to lose their cell wall? Was it a genetic condition? An environmental factor? Something was missing—a final piece of the puzzle that would come from an

---

i. Myco bacteria is also commonly found in people with *irritable bowel syndrome*, another intestinal disorder that doesn't feature the hallmark inflammation of Crohn's

unlikely source.

If you remember back to the study of sheep—where aluminum from the vaccines was tracked as it moved through their body—the places where the metal was most abundant were the lymph nodes. This makes sense because white blood cells transport aluminum around the body and lymph nodes tend to be gathering places for white blood cells. So no real surprise there—if your body has aluminum, we are likely to find it in the lymph nodes.

Your body contains a few areas of specialized lymph tissue that provide an early warning for your immune system. Some of this tissue surrounds your tonsils and adenoids and because they tend to hold a lot of white blood cells, they will also accumulate aluminum.[141]

Peyer's patches are kind of like the tonsils and adenoids of the gut— they help the immune system identify invaders in your intestine. Multiple studies have confirmed that aluminum tends to accumulate in this particular area.[142] This is significant because Peyer's patches are located in the terminal ileum—the same location from which Crohn's disease nearly always originates.

It would be an amazing coincidence that out of 28 feet of small and large intestine, the tiny area where Crohn's originates also contained a very special lymphatic component that tends to collect aluminum. The unlikelihood of such a coincidence has not gone unnoticed, and researchers have replicated how aluminum can cause the inflammation seen in Crohn's disease.[143] As scientists began to realize that aluminum was likely a causative factor in Crohn's, they begin to hone in on what might be causing the disease[144]—and even got tantalizing close, suggesting there was some relationship between aluminum and bacteria.[145]

Crohn's provides the perfect opportunity to understand the destructive nature of man-made disease. The inflammation caused by Crohn's is clearly visible in high resolution photographs taken during colonoscopies. Its spread can be easily tracked. It clearly has a microbial component to it—evidenced both by the way it spreads within the gut and how Crohn's inflammation can be transferred from one animal to another. It clearly has a metal toxicity component to it—evidenced both by studies that can create inflammation using aluminum and those that have found aluminum in the diseased intestinal tissue of animals.

What is actually causing Crohn's disease? A mix of metals, microbes and sometimes medicine. Aluminum—either from dietary intake or vaccines—accumulates in your lymph nodes, particularly the Peyer's patches located in your terminal ileum. The aluminum itself may be enough to cause painful inflammation, but for the long-running devastating effects that Crohn's is known for, another component is needed—possibly Mycobacterium avium paratuberculosis—the Myco bacteria.

Myco are hardy bacteria that anyone is likely to pick up from time to time as they can survive even the pasteurization of milk.[146] Like aluminum, the Myco bacteria—by themselves—may cause minor inflammation in the gut but your body's immune system will normally rid them with little fanfare.

Myco clearly have an affinity for the intestines, and in the presence of aluminum, things will take a turn for the worse. Aluminum increases your body's immune response to pathogens, and in the Peyer's patches—with a healthy supply of aluminum—an epic battle begins. The Mycobacterium invade the Peyer's patches where they encounter the aluminum. The nature of the metal changes Myco by stripping their cell wall, turning them into their intracellular version, a form which provides them with a new superpower—the ability to enter directly into white blood cells.

The bacteria begin to proliferate as they hide safely inside white blood cells, reproducing, growing in number, and weakening your body's ability to heal itself along the way. With fewer and fewer white blood cells functioning properly, your body begins to struggle to maintain control of the infection. The bacteria multiply in number and begin to spread into more of your intestine. Your body's natural response is to surround the bacteria and wall it off, much like it does with aluminum—an effect for which Crohn's is referred to as a *granulomatous* disease.

Normally, these granulomas would create productive inflammation and help reduce the infection, but in this abnormal state, they cause the disease to get worse. Many of the bacteria contained inside are intracellular and simply feed on the white blood cells that are arriving to help. The more help your body sends, the more easily they can replicate. The granulomas grow as the inflammation becomes worse. The crippling pains in your abdomen, the ulcerated tissue, and the increasing difficulty your body has absorbing nutrients from food—they are all clear signs your immune system is losing this battle.

In ulcerative colitis, the inflammation can be less aggressive than that seen in Crohn's disease and appears to be limited to the colon. Peyer's patches in the terminal ileum are not the only lymphoid tissue in the gut. Although they appear to have a special function in the immunology of the intestines, the rest of your gastrointestinal tract contains similar lymphoid tissue which may also accumulate aluminum.

It's possible the only difference between someone who has Crohn's disease and ulcerative colitis is where the bulk of metal ended up—maybe a random occurrence that has nothing to do with genetics or the environment. Perhaps the location of a minor infection when the aluminum was injected (or when an aluminum-containing granuloma elsewhere in your body ruptured) determined where the metal was drawn towards. If a significant amount of aluminum ends up in the Peyer's patches, you may stand a good chance of developing Crohn's disease at some point. Others might end up with more aluminum spread across the lymphoid-tissue of the colon, providing the intracellular bacteria with a foothold there.

Ulcerative colitis is less specifically associated with one bacteria, as studies have found anything from *Clostridium difficile*[147] to *Bacteroides vulgatus*.[148] The search for a particular bacteria and the characteristics of its spread and inflammation will help our understanding of how these diseases work. More importantly, we need to learn which antibiotics can negatively affect which bacteria. As with all things related to the immune system, the answer for one person may not hold true in another.

This is a very grim picture of what may be going on in Crohn's and ulcerative colitis. In a body free of metal or antibiotics, this sequence of events would never happen. The body could deal with the infection easily and would never develop the damage seen due to weeks, months, or years of constant inflammation. There is a reason the search for genetic answers to Crohn's has been elusive—it likely has little to do with genetics and much to do with the state of your immune system when you get a bacterial infection and the accumulation of metal in your body—specifically in the Peyer's patches.

Although the Myco bacteria is associated with Crohn's, I don't believe it is the only bacteria that can cause it. The different inflammation patterns of various Crohn's patients is undoubtedly due to many variables—possibly the idiosyncrasies of a particular bacteria, the genetic predispositions to inflammation, dietary influences, etc. But the mechanism is the same—metals or antibiotics give bacteria the ability to replicate within white blood cells and cause chronic inflammation your body is unable to stop.

A person completely free of metal—unfortunately an unlikely scenario in the modern age—who is given a dose of the wrong antibiotics might develop Crohn's disease or ulcerative colitis, though probably not to the extent we often see. A severely impaired immune system from stress or a recent illness might give just enough of an advantage to the bacteria to remain active for weeks.

Antibiotics have probably saved millions of lives in their short history and are not always avoidable. That leaves us with getting rid of the metal—for both prevention and healing. A few ideas regarding this and related topics are covered at the end of this book.

TUBEROUS SCLEROSIS COMPLEX

A rare genetic disorder called *tuberous sclerosis complex* (TSC) causes non-cancerous growths in different parts of your body—around your nose and eyes, for instance. It is not typically considered life threatening, but occasionally particular growths on the kidneys or brain can cause major problems. For this reason, patients with TSC are frequently monitored to make sure their growths do not need additional medical attention.

The reason I spent a lot of time looking at TSC despite its rarity is because it is considered by some to be the first identified cause of autism. Why? TSC can cause three types of growths in your brain. Two of the common ones are thought of as fairly innocuous, but the third, most rare type, can be also dangerous. The most common growths in a TSC brain are called cortical tubers. These small growths are present from birth and appear to calcify and harden over time, making them appear more prevalent on MRIs. Apparently, they do not grow much bigger over time.

Because autism is so prevalent in children with TSC, as often as

60% according to some,[149] the tuber growths in the brain were assumed to be the cause of autism. Consequently, there were a lot of studies done on TSC and its frequent association with the disorder.[150] It was thought that the locations and prevalence of these cortical tubers might unlock the mysteries of autism in children without the TSC diagnosis.

Unfortunately, these studies did not correlate well with the behaviors parents were seeing. It was thought that tubers might affect the temporal lobe, for instance—a part of the brain responsible for processing speech and facial recognition—but there were children that exhibited this behavior and showed no growths in that area of their brain.

After having taken a serious look at possible connections, progress has stalled. According to research published by the excellent Tuberous Sclerosis Alliance,[i] "it is now clear that the presence of cortical tubers is not sufficient on its own to produce ASD (autism spectrum disorder)."[151]

Similarly, the cortical tubers were also assumed to be the cause of epilepsy, present in as many as 90% of children with TSC, but research has failed to find a specific connection. Confounding research into this area: there are TSC patients with no tubers who still have seizures, and children with significant tuber growths with no seizures. And finally, some people seem to outgrow their seizures, leading medicine-free lives as adults, where as children, medication was the only thing that could help. The connections between TSC, epilepsy and autism seemed promising initially, but have turned up little hope for prevention.

Tuberous Sclerosis was one of the first diseases I begin researching years ago. As the connection between inflammation and the way metals move around the body began to materialize, I felt like the link with TSC and with autism would become clear to me. It took a while, but it

i. For such a rare disease, the professionalism of their work and amount of research this organization has generated is incredible.

finally happened.

Because of recent scientific research, I understood that aluminum, a potent neurotoxin, did not move around your body randomly, but was transported to specific areas via signaling requests for help by your immune system. So given what I knew about triggers—infection, pregnancy, exertion and stress—I struggled to understand what might cause one of these triggers in tuberous sclerosis.

The answer would came out of nowhere one day as I read through some random forum postings on TSC. A terrified mother had just seen her baby's MRI:

> "When my son was born they did an MRI and found that he has lots of random tumors in his brain. They told me that they would keep developing but how is this possible? If they keep developing...would he run out of room for his brain to work properly? This scares me. there's only so much room in his little head, im so scared to think about the future, Are there any parents with kids who have had TSC since birth and are older and are doing fine? Please give me some answers. Thank you"

I shudder to think of what parents who've experienced this must have felt. A few people chimed in to offer support, and one of them, clearly an experienced parent with scientific knowledge, attempted to explain the good and the bad about what she had seen:

> "So SEN and tubers develop as the brain develops but then stay about the same size … You might think of the SEN and cortical tubers as abnormal tissue, like scar tissue. A scar is still skin tissue, it is not a tumor getting bigger, however it is not made of the right kind of cells to look or act like the surrounding tissue."[152]

* * *

I immediately thought back to the "BB" under my wife's scar and our friend's lump under her scar. Both of them had occurred within a few weeks of receiving an injection of aluminum. I was fairly certain this person had just provided a clue for the plausible explanation I had been looking for.

The growths in TSC are like tiny little scars, dispersed throughout your brain. Like my wife's post-op scar, they don't hurt. They're not uncomfortable and yet, your body knows the difference. It's not fooled —not in the least. It will keep a vigilant watch on these areas, sending white blood cells for help, just in case. If my theory is correct, even a skinned knee you got when you were four years old could still be receiving extra attention from your immune system ninety years from now.

And so it might be with tuberous sclerosis. The growths are abnormalities due to a failure to adequately suppress cell growth. They may be present from the time someone is 8 cells big, but even so, the immune system can detect they are not supposed to be there. Their presence triggers immune activation, and white blood cells are summoned to these areas for help. Unfortunately, these white blood cells are likely to contain aluminum—a neurotoxin that can cause problems in tiny amounts.

Removing these areas of growths is likely to show improvement in seizures, convincing surgeons they determined the correct cause. I propose it's not the growths themselves causing the problem but the toxin they have summoned—it's not the removal of tubers that stop the seizures, but the removal of the metal around them. The ability for aluminum to disguise itself is maddening.

ZIKA

In the fall of 2015, troubling reports began to surface in the Northeastern sections of Brazil. Doctors were seeing an increase in the number of babies born with undersized heads, a phenomenon called *microcephaly*. As the months passed, it became clear that something had happened—there was a massive spike in the number of microcephaly cases, an absolutely heartbreaking thing to see on the news. Besides the obvious physical deformity, babies born in this condition would likely suffer neurological delays and learning disabilities. Health officials frantically searched for answers as to why this was happening. Despite locals pointing to the recent release of genetically modified mosquitoes or the aggressive pesticide spraying they had been recently subjected to, the authorities were sure they had found the cause. It was a relatively unknown illness that had recently been introduced into the country – a microbe transmitted by mosquito bite called the *Zika virus*.

A year or so earlier, the World Health Organization had botched its response to the Ebola outbreak in Africa, and amidst rumors of its increasing irrelevance in a modern world of nimble, efficient charities like the Bill & Melinda Gates Foundation, it would use its response to the Zika crisis as a show of force and relevancy. With all hands on deck, the WHO's response was indeed massive. Government agencies from around the world were involved. There were outlandish requests for research and funding. Continual press conferences and media blitzes put the threat of Zika onto the front page of nearly every news outlet and television broadcast in the world. Billions of dollars of funding were being mobilized to understand this disaster and develop vaccines to prevent it.

Zika was a new threat, particularly to pregnant women, the authorities repeated over and over. Apparently even their sexual partners could transmit the virus to them and harm their fetus. Athletes, who had trained their entire lives to compete in the 2016 Summer Olympics, pulled out of competition rather than risk harming their future offspring. Health authorities as far away as the United States began dropping pesticides over large cities—with chemicals that were known to cause birth defects themselves—in an attempt to control the outbreak. Scientific papers and press releases were rushed into publication: "CDC Concludes Zika Causes Microcephaly and Other Birth Defects."[153] It was possibly the most widespread, expensive, pro-active response to a pathogenic threat since polio.

Except there was problem—Brazil and other countries with active Zika infections continued into 2016, but the cases of microcephaly did not. The dire predictions of health officials, understandably frazzled by the hysterical response from the WHO, did not come to pass. The birth defects returned to their previous levels. Microcephaly and other anomalies were now being actively monitored—every infant head carefully measured—throughout most of South America and beyond.

Despite the hyper vigilance of the medical community and Zika infections continuing to happen, even amongst pregnant women, the birth defects were decreasing. Zika infections were still occurring, and the science was clear—Zika infections caused microcephaly. Even some of the media, which breathlessly relayed every dire warning and bullet-point from the WHO, began asking the question—what happened? "Why Didn't Zika Cause A Surge In Microcephaly in 2016?"[154] an NPR reporter asked a few health officials, including Christopher Dye, an obviously uncomfortable Ebola Team Lead from the World Health Organization.

Dye suggests that perhaps they had vastly miscounted the number of actual Zika infections in Brazil, mistaking them for another virus called *chikungunya*, an answer the plucky reporter was obviously not impressed with. "Now for this theory to hold true," she responded, "we're talking about thousands of Zika cases being mistaken for a totally different virus that's not even closely related to Zika. Could this really happen?"

No, it could not have happened. But I think I know what did happen, and the answer only recently became clear to me as the mechanisms by which metals and microbes harm fell into place.

I had watched the Zika story closely ever since it broke, trying to make sense of what had happened. The massive WHO response baffled me until I realized they were covering for their Ebola missteps. But the problem *was* horrifying—Zika infections seemed to be growing and health officials were understandably concerned.

As I poured through the science surrounding Zika research, two papers stood out. First, the virus has an affinity for neural stem cells.[155] Neural stem cells are important to the development of not just the brain, but the entire central nervous system, possibly even the peripheral nervous system, as they can "self-renew" and form into the many different specialized cells required for its function.

Secondly, the virus had apparently mutated in some form to cause a more infectious strain sometime before a small 2013 outbreak in French Polynesia.[156] A more infectious strain might provide a cause for the recent Zika outbreaks, as it apparently made its way into the Americas around 2014. The research I found might explain why there were more Zika infections, and they might explain how Zika might cause neurological development problems, but they didn't explain the sudden spike in 2015, nor the sudden disappearance in 2016.

I was at a dead end—until I remembered the 2014 technical report that had been issued nationwide by the Brazilian Health Department's Immunization Division.[i] In October 2014, Brazilian health officials issued a new decree—Pertussis, also known as Whooping Cough, was shaping up to be a big problem, and they were recommending the shot be given for all pregnant women. But there was an ominous part of the bulletin that should have concerned any physician reading it—for any woman not vaccinated previously for pertussis, the bulletin recommended:

> *"Administer the first two doses of dT and the last dose of dTpa between the 27th and preferably up to the 36th week of gestation."*[157]

They were recommending pregnant women receive up to three doses of this shot, containing up to .4 mg of aluminum each. The doctors, it would appear, took the memo seriously. PBS Frontline did an interview with several mothers in Brazil whose babies had developed microcephaly:

> *"Ederlanha, an 18-year-old mother of a child recently diagnosed with microcephaly, is inclined to believe vaccines may be the problem. She says she never had symptoms of Zika, but*

---

i. This memo has been removed from the internet but can be found via archive.org and translated online. I have included a link to my personal translation of the document in the endnotes.

she did receive a shot from her public health clinic every month of her pregnancy. As she waited for an appointment at the public hospital in Recife, she tried to soothe her fussing baby, but said she couldn't recall exactly what the shots were for.[158]

We can only hope she didn't actually receive a vaccine every month of her pregnancy, but from the unease of other mothers around this time and area, you can tell there were a lot of them. She also doesn't recall having anything resembling a Zika infection at all, not surprising given the innocuous nature of the virus.

Knowing that most of these 2015 microcephaly cases appeared in a specific region of Brazil, amongst some of the poorest mothers in that area, one could see how their vaccination status might fall into the "unknown" category. It's also not hard to imagine a recently inspired doctor wanting to be extra-sure the poor mother's baby wouldn't have to suffer a Pertussis infection and erring on the "safe" side by administering a three-shot course of injections—just in case. Hopefully the 18-year old Ederlanha's memory is faulty and they stopped at three.

What do I think happened? I believe that Zika had recently surfaced in a very particular area—northeastern Brazil in 2014. It was relatively unknown to South America until this time. In the other areas of the world with previous infections, Zika had been an innocuous virus that wasn't associated with microcephaly.[ii] It was a new disease vector, and was fanning out just like you might expect any other infection to spread. Zika turns out to be a peculiar infection because it does appear to cause inflammation in the fetal brain—something the maternal and fetal immune system apparently can cope with under normal circumstances—as evidenced by a lack of birth defects associated with Zika more often than not.

---

ii. An impossibly small study of an outbreak in French Polynesia did make this association within a 2013-2014 outbreak.

It has been argued that vaccines have not been adequately safety tested on pregnant women. Even if they were, we can be sure the safety tests would not have permitted administering 3 or more doses during one pregnancy. The 2014 Brazilian memo came at the worst possible time for some. It was a national roll-out and there were undoubtedly mothers across the country that received multiple doses of the TDaP vaccine during their pregnancy. The outcomes of those pregnancies is unknown.

But for a very unlucky group of women—those who received multiple injections of aluminum and got a Zika infection at the same time, the outcome was not going to be good. From what we know about the infection, it is likely to have created inflammation in the neural stem cells of the fetal brain. Again—with a properly functioning immune system, most babies could evidently make it through unscathed. However, with their white blood cells flush with aluminum, it's unsurprising that when these poor children's immune systems asked for help, they received a neurotoxic response.

The technical memo is now gone from the Brazilian Health Department's site—it has completely disappeared and I had to use special tools to find an archived version. There is no reference to this program or any recommendations that I can find regarding pregnant women and this vaccine. And in a final note of irony, I realized the memo was released in October 2014. Exactly ten months later, in August of 2015, the first cases of microcephaly began to appear. It would seem that Zika, without the aluminum injections, is an innocuous disease. Apparently the Brazilian health officials who have removed all references to this health memo would agree, even if they don't fully understand what happened.

CHRONIC TRAUMATIC ENCEPHALOPATHY

I first heard of *chronic traumatic encephalopathy* (CTE) soon after NFL player Junior Seau killed himself at 43 years old. I had been a fan of his, watching him play at the San Diego Chargers for years, then watching him finish out his career with the New England Patriots.

Something seemed amiss when in 2010 he crashed his SUV, falling 100 feet over a cliff, just hours after he had been arrested for domestic violence. He claimed to have fallen asleep while driving, but for many who had followed his career, a sense of foreboding took over. Something was wrong, but no one knew why.

Seau stayed out of the news for the most part, until on May 2, 2012, when his girlfriend found him dead from a gunshot wound to his chest. He had killed himself, and the sports world was shocked. There wasn't any substance abuse problems, as far as I knew. He was active in charity organizations and besides the domestic violence charge preceding his car crash, I didn't remember him having any criminal record.

Behind the scenes, Seau was struggling terribly. He had battled insomnia for over seven years, and a case was brought against the doctor prescribing him Ambien, claiming he had ignored the warning signs of depression and suicidal thought.[159]

A few months later, Seau's family suggested that examination of his brain tissue revealed evidence of CTE—trauma consistent with someone suffering repeated head injuries. It was another case of a young, otherwise healthy athlete who began suffering from extreme depression and behavior problems, only to ultimately end their life as modern medicine never seemed to offer any help.

I made note of an interesting piece of information: Seau had no reported history of concussions. His wife mentioned that he had sustained concussions during his career, but the official record showed none.

I began to read through the various stories from "Legacy Donors" on the Concussion Legacy Foundation website. These were heartbreaking tales, often of very young athletes, stricken down in the prime of their life by unexplainable depression, anxiety and behavioral problems that were untreatable and often became so debilitating suicide seemed the only way out.

These stories struck me as odd—something new was going on. This wasn't "one too many concussions" for a young kid. If anything, helmets had gotten bigger over the last 30 years. Coaches and parents have become more wary. Kid's soccer leagues won't let them head the ball, and some players have elected to wear a padded headband, just in case.

Across the board, sports should have become more safe, but people have become so wary of this new disease that recently, a twenty-four year old NFL player named Chris Borland walked away from a stellar career and massive paycheck rather than continue the risk of the debilitating effects of CTE.

Even at the professional level, helmets were considered optional in football until the late 1930s. Hockey players rarely wore them until the 1970s. And yet, these players, who must have sustained more head trauma than the technologically advanced and watched-over players of today receive, seemed to have little evidence of anything resembling CTE.

According to the Concussion Legacy Foundation, it's not the concussions that are necessarily the main problem—the biggest concern is what they call the subconcussive impacts. Junior Seau's lack of officially recognized concussions was not an anomaly. Many of the people featured on the CTE website had very few, if any, concussions in their young careers.

Research organizations have worked together by employing tiny measurement devices tucked into helmets, around necks, and even into mouth guards to measure and analyze the impacts of high-contact sports. They have determined that concussions—massive head trauma likely to knock you unconscious—is not necessary to develop CTE. It is multiple smaller hits to the head—the subconcussive impacts—which over time seem to cause more of a problem.

Two seemingly insignificant bits of information led me to believe I understood what was actually causing CTE. In the beginning of NFL football games, they will always go through the team lineups, showing headshots of each person playing in the game. I had noticed how common strabismus was amongst these players, but was especially struck when I looked through pictures of young men who had died from CTE related issues. Many of them showed signs of facial palsy—crooked smiles, misaligned eyes. Seeing it on the faces of these young men who had died in their youth gave me added urgency in understanding what had happened to them.

The second clue emerged as I was going through some literature on the pathological findings of CTE. Researchers were struck by the similarities between CTE brains and those of people that had died of Alzheimer's disease. In fact, when I began to look at the PET scans and cross sections of actual brain tissue, they looked identical. With a couple of CTE and Alzheimer's brains in a lineup, even an expert would be hard pressed to pick out which was which. How could this be? Alzheimer's, a disease of the elderly, causing forgetfulness, confusion, the inability to recognize common things. And CTE, a disease typically found in athletes that participated in full contact sports. Young, healthy—with behavioral issues and suicidal thoughts. But there was also cognitive impairment. Short-term memory loss. Difficulty carrying out tasks. Overlap, between Alzheimer's and CTE. And I was beginning to think I might know why.

THE ORIGINAL ALZHEIMER'S DISEASE

"There is no word in the English language more deserving of a precise definition than madness..."

– John Haslam

Where was Alzheimer's disease two hundred years ago? Like the search for autoimmune disease, I believed that if medicinal metals were the cause of our modern neurological woes, then we should see them in the early 1800s, if only on a limited scale. And so, Alzheimer's, or something like it, should be floating around the literature, waiting to be recognized.

It was not hard to find. *General Paralysis of the Insane*, or GPI, is believed to have first been mentioned by John Haslam in an 1809 book called "Observations on Madness and Melancholy." Haslam and other doctors of the time were becoming concerned with an increase in *insanity*, and he felt compelled to write about what he was seeing.

* * *

"Paralytic affections are a much more frequent cause of insanity than has been commonly supposed, and they are also a very common effect of madness… These patients usually bear marks of such affection, independently of their insanity: the speech is impeded, and the mouth is drawn aside; an arm, or leg, is more or less deprived of its capability of being moved by the will, and in most of them the memory is particularly impaired."[160]

One hundred years later in 1913, as the disease had become prevalent, a more nuanced description was made by one of the world's preeminent psychiatrists, Emil Kraepelin:

"The patient is absent-minded, inattentive, does not grasp events transpiring about him with accustomed clearness. He does not notice details, loses the drift in a conversation and fails to hear questions asked him or answers those directed to others. He mistakes persons and objects, overlooks important circumstances or changes, which would not have escaped him before; loses himself among familiar surroundings. I remember a man who suddenly, one day, was unable to find his place of work where he had been regularly employed."[161]

Kraepelin was describing a neurological phenomenon that had rarely been seen. In the past, patients typically had problems with long-term memory, but in these new cases, "the patient forgets, unlike the ordinary memory relations, the more recent happenings."[162] An area of the brain called the hippocampus prepares short term memories for long-term storage, a common deficiency in Alzheimer's disease. Other similarities are present like *echolalia*[i] and a lack of self-restraint, as

---

i. Repeating words and phrases that are said to you.

evidenced by grabbing someone else's food or belongings.

I will spare you the gory details, but autopsies of GPI brains left little doubt as to why they had died. Whereas Alzheimer's or Parkinson's might require a microscope to spot the problem, the discoloration, fluid and deformation in GPI cranial tissue was unmistakably damaged. Although most modern readers will have never even heard of GPI, it was inevitably fatal and was the 7th leading cause of death in New York State, even as late as 1914,[163] almost 15 years after the discovery of Alzheimer's.[ii]

There was a common thread that doctors initially missed: everyone with GPI had been infected with syphilis at one point. Until penicillin was available in 1942, syphilis was invariably treated aggressively with mercury. Anyone who had become infected with the disease would likely develop mercury poisoning of some kind—if they hoped to live. The mercury did work at some level, so "A night with Venus, a lifetime with Mercury" became a popular saying of the day.

The bacteria that causes syphilis, *Treponema pallidum*, has a particularly affinity for brain tissue. Though syphilis is a sexually transmitted infection, the bacteria can, over the course of 10 to 20 years, begin to make their way to the brain. The obvious question— were bacteria actually causing the symptoms of GPI, or were they merely causing the neurological inflammation that ended up signaling mercury into the brain? The mechanism of Alzheimer's disease would prove to offer a remarkable answer to its GPI predecessor.

---

ii. Alzheimer's is currently the 6th leading cause of death in the U.S.

ALZHEIMER'S DISEASE

"I remember the first time I realized something was really wrong," a woman told me, recounting the story of her mother's decline.

"We'd gone home for Thanksgiving and I was playing in the backyard with the kids to give her a break. She needed some space—I could tell. Holidays with out-of-town family is stressful, kids are loud, I get it. I could tell it was getting to her."

Like so many elderly people and their families and caregivers, this woman's story would mirror the painful descent they had seen. One of her kids wandered into the flowerbed in the center of the backyard.

"Mom tore out onto the porch and started screaming at him. She said words none of us had ever heard her say. I ran onto the porch and tried to calm her down and get her back inside. She'd turned into someone—something I'd never, ever seen in her. I was shaking it scared me so bad."

After getting her mother some water, she went back outside to calm her shocked children.

"I didn't know what to say to them. It was just—so completely out of left field. No one in our family screams or talks like that. They'd never seen it before."

Over the following weeks, this woman's awareness of something happening to her mother grew, and other symptoms she had chalked up to old age began to take on a new significance—forgotten birthdays, late power bill notices on the kitchen counter—things she would have never done previously.

"A few months later as we spoke on the phone, I asked her about the Thanksgiving incident. She had no idea—no memory of it happening. We were already concerned at that point, obviously, but when she started forgetting names of people, and one time it was my brother's name—that was when I knew it had gotten really bad."

Another common refrain—waiting things out, hoping that somehow their loved ones wouldn't get worse.

"I don't know what took us so long. I lived out of town, and my brother had never been that involved. Why it took two years of this to finally start looking for help—I don't know. It's awkward, I guess."

The woman talked about two of the doctor appointments she had gone to, her mom reluctantly attending one of them.

"They made it seem normal, like this was just part of the aging process. I'm old enough to remember my great-grandmother, plus three of my grand-parents. None of them went through this. My grandmother was forgetful at the end, but she was 92 years old. She was happy. She was still herself. What happened to my mom wasn't just getting old—it was something different. She was 68 when we first noticed it. She made it to 73."

Patient zero, the first Alzheimer's patient, was Auguste Deter. She was fifty-one years old in 1901 when she was admitted to a hospital and seen by Alois Alzheimer for the strange constellation of neurological symptoms she exhibited: Waking up in the middle of the night, screaming. Memory problems. Difficulty reading and writing. Disorientation.

Alzheimer would follow this woman's decline until her death almost six years later. He did a thorough examination of her brain and described two abnormalities—*neurofibrillary tangles* and *amyloid plaques*—anomalies which (in addition to the loss of brain mass) are still the trademark characteristics of the disease today.

Since then, hundreds of millions of dollars of research have been poured into understanding the causes of this horrible disease. While our appreciation of the way in which the tangles and plaques are formed has grown, the "why" has so far been elusive. Treatments are limited and at this point, a cure seems but a remote possibility. In the meantime, prevalence has grown so much so that Alzheimer's disease is now the 6th leading cause of death in the United States,[164] and familial Alzheimer's (early-onset Alzheimer's) seems to be on the rise.

What is causing this illness? Is it, like many insist with autism, an overlooked set of symptoms that has always existed amongst our population? Or is it a relatively new phenomenon whose rising rates we should legitimately be concerned with? Could my theories describe a plausible mechanism for the cause of Alzheimer's disease?

Besides the tangles and plaques, another hallmark of Alzheimer's disease is chronic inflammation.[165] Whether this inflammation is a response to some other damage or possibly the cause of it is hotly debated.[166] Similar to many other diseases like rheumatoid arthritis or even asthma, systemic infections and the resulting inflammation clearly seem to exacerbate their symptoms.[167] Interestingly, seniors who were on anti-inflammatory medicine seemed to have a lower rate of Alzheimer's. And it would appear that it's not only the damaged brains of Alzheimer patients that resemble CTE (Chronic Traumatic Encephalopathy) but the risk factors as well: traumatic brain injury is a common precursor[168] to Alzheimer's disease.

This line of research regarding the cause of Alzheimer's didn't catch my attention until I began to follow the studies of scientists from Keele University who had begun to perfect methods of quantifying the amount aluminum in tissue samples, something which had previously been very difficult.

When Dr. Christopher Exley, a scientist who had spent most of his career understanding the toxicity of aluminum, began to find alarming levels of the metal in the brain tissue of people who had died of Alzheimer's, there was little response from the disease's community. No calls for more research and few media appearances for the team. The website of the leading charity, Alzheimer's Association, went even further, publishing a note of assurance to their members that "studies have failed to confirm any role for aluminum in causing Alzheimer's. Experts today focus on other areas of research, and few believe that everyday sources of aluminum pose any threat."[169] This is an increasingly difficult statement to claim, yet they still have it posted on their website today.

Exley and his team would go on to measure aluminum in the brains of donors who had died of early-onset Alzheimer's.[170] They would find some of the highest ever measured concentrations of aluminum in human brain tissue.[i] Others would be able to recreate the symptoms of Alzheimer's disease in animal models simply by increasing the aluminum in their diets.[171] Scientists also demonstrated how aluminum can damage the hippocampus, that part of the brain responsible for converting short-term memories into long-term ones,[172] a common symptom of Alzheimer's disease.

As always, many would cling to the search for a genetic answer. It certainly factors into the equation, as some populations[173] such as those

---

i. A seemingly impossible amount of aluminum that several months later was easily surpassed when they measured the brain tissue of autistic donors.

with Down's syndrome absorb more aluminum from their digestive tract,[174] but regardless, the environmental levels of the metal would have to be considered to have reached a tipping point, given recent increases in the disease.

With CTE, there is an obvious cause of inflammation. With Alzheimer's, it is less clear. Could it be possible that intracellular bacteria are the source of chronic inflammation in the brain? Intracellular bacteria reproduce inside white blood cells and are very difficult for your body's immune system to kill off. Could aluminum and/or possibly antibiotics create the vicious circle of chronic inflammation that slowly draws any injected or dietary metals into the brain?

Unfortunately, it is not only possible, I believe it's likely. A 2015 meta-analysis from the Journal of Alzheimer's disease found there was over a 10-fold increase in Alzheimer's disease when the presence of spirochetal infection was detected—a discovery that makes Alzheimer's look just like its sibling from yesteryear, GPI. There was a 5-fold increase in the occurrence of Alzheimer's disease when *Chlamydophila pneumoniae* infections were detected.[175] C. pneumoniae are often the cause of pneumonia in the elderly. They are spread through the air and easily caught. Most infections are dealt with quickly by the immune system, but in the presence of aluminum and/or antibiotics, they could possibly survive for months, even years, as a low-grade infection.

A disturbing study even went so far as to show how these bacteria, because of their lack of cell wall, are able to sneak past the blood brain barrier.[176] The inflammation caused by long running infections could easily explain why so much aluminum is found in the brains of Alzheimer's patients. The inflammation brings the aluminum. The aluminum causes more bacteria to lose their cell wall, preventing the immune system from ever getting ahead. It's a perfect storm of neurodegenerative disease.

* * *

The grave concerns of the Keele scientist could not be masked when in June of 2017, an editorial was published in the Journal of Alzheimer's Disease Reports entitled "Aluminum Should Now Be Considered a Primary Etiological Factor in Alzheimer's Disease."[177] Exley, arguably the preeminent scholar on aluminum toxicity, attempted to sound the alarm on Alzheimer's and aluminum in the strongest possible way, but like the reactions many Autism organizations have had to recent scientific research, the Alzheimer charities responded with silence or condemnation.

While Alzheimer's may have typically arisen in the later years of life due to a very gradual accumulation of dietary aluminum, the amount of environmental aluminum present in today's children—due to the numerous vaccines they receive—points to the likelihood we will see a massive increase in the numbers of early-onset Alzheimer's in the coming decades. This is to say nothing of the athletes, soldiers and other activities that are predisposed to create cranial inflammation. Given the remarkably similar appearance of Alzheimer's and CTE damaged brains, and knowing that they both share a common denominator in chronic inflammation, it seems that it will only be a matter of time before aluminum is also implicated in the growing debate about concussion-related disease.

And the overlap continues beyond Alzheimer's and CTE into Parkinson's and other forms of dementia. Creating an explicit diagnosis that firmly places someone in the Alzheimer's or Parkinson's bucket can be difficult. There are similarities and commonalities that change from one person to the next and one day to the next. We may one day realize that—similar to autism—all of these forms of dementia lie within the same broad spectrum. Perhaps the Autism and Dementia spectrums themselves will later merge.

The inevitable suggestion will be to test CTE brains for aluminum.

There is a growing brain bank of donors for research, and it would only make sense to run tests on these brains to check for elevated aluminum levels. I am not sure if this is true, but I believe that the materials in which these particular brains have been preserved contains aluminum and will make testing difficult. It is recommended that CTE-related brain banks begin storing their donor tissue in a different format that allows for accurate testing of aluminum levels.

If your child is fully-vaccinated and is playing full-contact sports like football, soccer, lacrosse or hockey, you may want to look into this issue more deeply. As a reminder, these are unproven theories I am proposing, and I wouldn't force your child to quit sports because of this one thing. However, from what we know about Alzheimer's and its similarities with CTE, I would do everything I could to minimize my children's exposure to even mild brain trauma.

A statement in the editorial by Exley would echo the exact sentiment expressed by the woman at the beginning of this chapter.

"Alzheimer's disease," he wrote, "is not an inevitable consequence of aging in the absence of a brain burden of aluminum."[178]

Or as the woman would put it, "What happened to my mom wasn't just getting old—it was something different."

PANDAS

There is no clearer indication of a child suffering the effects of chronic inflammation than the symptoms seen with *Pediatric Autoimmune Neuropsychiatric Disorder Associated with Strep* (PANDAS) or *Pediatric Acute-onset Neuropsychiatric Syndrome* (PANS)[i]. This illness often comes on after an infection and can change a completely healthy, happy child into a raging tempest of sensory-overloaded anxiety. They may show improvements, only to have the symptoms return with another illness. And illness—sinus infections, ear infections or colds—all seem very common in children with PANDAS.

During an episode—what parents of children with PANDAS call a *flare*—children might experience meltdowns, full-body tics, sensory issues, OCD, anger, mood changes, destructive and self-injurious behavior (SIB). It's not unheard of to see children clawing at their face until they draw blood, crying in pain and confusion the whole time.

---

i. I will use PANDAS for brevity.

Just a hundred years ago, parents of a child that experienced these dramatic changes would not have sent for the doctor, but a priest. They would have assumed their previously angelic son or daughter had become possessed by an evil spirit. In our modern age, we may laugh at such an unenlightened response, but the truth is even the best doctors often fair no better with their treatment than an exorcist might.

Beyond the extreme nature of the flares, one of the things that makes PANDAS so difficult is the children are often just old enough to tell their parents they're sorry. They realize that something is not right with them. If it were a one or two year old, their verbal skills might not give them the ability to convey this emotion. When they are four years and up, they are often perfectly capable of expressing confusion about their behavior—an absolutely heartbreaking confession for any parent to deal with.

Stories of parents trying to understand what is going wrong with their children are infuriating. They're often told their children will grow out of these behaviors—that they are normal outbursts for "defiant" children. They are told their child may not be getting enough sleep or the parents need to learn how to mete out more discipline.

But often both parent *and* child know better – they can tell that something is very wrong. After months, sometimes years of suffering, they may finally get a diagnosis of PANDAS or PANS. A doctor may suggest a tonsillectomy—the surgery physicians have been turning to when all else fails for over one hundred years. During prep for the surgery, they notice the child has signs of an infection and they test for strep, which is positive. The parents will often have had no idea their child had an infection as they showed no outward signs of it.

After the surgery, their child is put on an antibiotic for the strep infection. Miraculously, their symptoms improve. Their angel child is back. No OCD. No outbursts—as if the whole thing had been a bad dream. But a few weeks after the antibiotic is stopped, the nightmare returns as the manic episodes and behavioral problems come back worse than ever. Steroids are tried and give the parents and child a brief respite from their suffering—but their effects are limited. More antibiotics are tried, this time intravenously with a *PIC line*. Again, symptoms improve for a bit but return with a vengeance.

What is going on with these poor children? Parts of their brain have become inflamed with infection, and their immune systems are being made powerless to help, wrecked by metals and antibiotic use.

If you go back through many of the other neurodegenerative disorders we've looked at, you will see many of the signs of PANDAS. Sensory disorders such as refusing to eat or constantly dilated pupils due to a dysfunctioning thalamus. Behavioral disorders such as SIBs and destroying things due to the perpetual fight-or-flight cortisol dump from a dysfunctioning hypothalamic-pituitary axis. The specific parts of the brain affected by these infections will vary from person to person and bacteria to bacteria.

In a normal immune system, the body could get ahead of the infections before the inflammation that can cause this behavior ever surfaced. When these children get an infection, especially if they have been recently injected with aluminum-containing vaccines, it creates a metal and microbe cascade that can be made worse by the addition of antibiotics.

During the initial infection, strep or otherwise, part of the inflammation occurs in their brain. In a body full of metal, this otherwise trivial infection kicks off a chain of events that leads to serious problems. The inflammation draws aluminum to the site, possibly damaging parts of the brain. The aluminum also aids the bacteria in transforming into their intracellular form, making them very difficult to detect by the immune system. While these intracellular bacteria are replicating inside the white blood cells, they are suppressing the immune system and creating the stage for chronic infection.

After the physician suspects that something is actually wrong, they may prescribe a penicillin antibiotic which like the metal, can turn some bacteria into a form that is very difficult for the body to get rid of. Other types of bacteria, may sense they are being challenged and transform into other forms like cysts or band together in *biofilms* to protect themselves. As a result, the inflammation decreases and both child and parent experience what feels like a miracle of healing.

Once the antibiotic is stopped, the intracellular bacteria abandon their cyst-like structures, creating many more copies of themselves in the process—an unfortunate event which can create more neurological inflammation. The symptoms come raging back, worse than ever. Both parent and doctor are completely confused at the inability of the antibiotic to have any lasting effect on the child's health.

The most destructive trait of PANDAS is the massive cortisol release. The constant state of extreme anxiety—obviously visible in the child's behavior—diverts all resources away from their immune system and could explain why PANDAS children are constantly getting sick. It could also explain why so many PANDAS children have infections discovered by luck rather than by symptom—their horribly suppressed immune system doesn't have enough energy to even manifest a cough or runny nose.

The techniques mentioned in the healing and recovery chapter should help with PANDAS. Of all the disorders mentioned in this book, the rise and fall of PANDAS symptoms—with infection, the temporary abatement of symptoms with antibiotic use, only to return much worse—all clearly point to a brain that is suffering from chronic inflammation and an immune system that is unable to help. While metals certainly play a part of PANDAS, the dramatic rise and fall of symptoms point to intense bacterial inflammation.

CHRONIC FATIGUE SYNDROME

Fibromyalgia and chronic fatigue syndrome (CFS)[i] clearly demonstrate the problems you will encounter when thinking of modern disease within the framework of classical medicine. The overlap between the two conditions can make it difficult for doctors who are trying to make an explicit diagnosis.

For some people, there may appear to be no overlap at all. They may exhibit the symptoms of fibromyalgia and have a family member with CFS and not share a single symptom. Others may have the debilitating fatigue of CFS but suffer "fibro-fog" cognitive impairment and irritable bowel syndrome occasionally.

If you look at these conditions through the lens we have created in understanding man-made disease, the overlap will begin to make sense. According to the theories laid out in this book, man-made illnesses are either due to acute neuron damage from metal toxicity or the chronic inflammation from long-running bacterial infections

---

i. Also referred to as myalgic encephalomyelitis or ME in some countries.

enabled by metals and/or antibiotics. I believe that the core symptoms of both fibromyalgia and CFS arise from dysfunction in the *thalamus* and *hypothalamus* of the brain due to a persistent low-grade bacterial infection. If the inflammation is chiefly in the thalamus, you will predominantly experience symptoms of fibromyalgia. If the inflammation is predominantly in the hypothalamus, you will experience the effects of chronic fatigue syndrome.

The thalamus and hypothalamus are directly beside each other and their proximity is the reason why many people experience symptoms of both illnesses. As the inflammation fluctuates between these two adjacent structures, you may notice an increase in fatigue or an increase in pain. Although people could be experiencing inflammation due to a variety of bacteria, for a particular person, their suffering is most likely due to a single infection in their brain—one cause for both problems.

The onset of both disorders is typically associated with either a serious illness such as mono or a stressful, traumatic event—like a car accident. Due to subsequent immune activation[ii], I believe that white-blood cells containing metals are drawn to that area of your brain. They might cause neuronal damage initially, but their long-term effects may be much worse. If you were administered antibiotics during this time, the inflammation from your initial sickness could have made the blood-brain-barrier more permeable, allowing both the antibiotic and possibly a bacterial infection to pass inside.

Either way, your body recovered from the initial infection, perhaps the Epstein-Barre virus, but a bacterial invader found a weak point in your body—the aluminum that accumulated around your thalamus or hypothalamus. The aluminum caused the bacteria to lose its cell wall, allowing it to replicate inside your white blood cells. Your immune system became suppressed from losing massive numbers of white

---

ii. Look up the hypothalamic–pituitary–adrenal axis, or HPA for an explanation of the stress response.

blood cells to intracellular bacteria replication and couldn't mount a sustained attack to kill them. A month or two after the initial mono infection cleared, weeks of inflammation from this new bacterial infection began to show their effects.

If you experienced this sequence of events and your chronic infection is damaging the hypothalamus, you may begin to encounter crippling tiredness. The reason we know this is interesting. In the early 1900s, research was carried out to understand the nature of muscles, exercise and fatigue. Based on the results of these studies, a century of erroneous thinking emerged—the heart was the limiting factor in physical output. Because of this, it was thought that elite-level athletes had better hearts that could pump harder for longer, allowing them to continue performing at their peak while others began to fade.

It's become obvious this can't be the sole determining factor. Athletes will often perform at levels during competition they are unable to achieve in practice, despite their best attempts. Runners at the end of a close race can often summon reserves for a last push when seconds earlier they felt as if they had no energy left. I'm reminded of the Tour de France, a grueling bicycle race through thousands of miles of Europe, which has been said to be a contest in pain management as much as it is cycling.

Studies have looked within fatigued muscle tissue for metabolites and other markers of tiredness but have found little.[179] It has long been thought that an accumulation of lactic acid from exertion was triggering pain within the muscles but it appears that fatigue can set in long before the majority of your muscle fibers have been used. A study done in 2004 determined that only 35% to 50% of skeletal muscle mass is employed during active exercise.[180] As muscle fatigue sets in, the brain can recruit additional muscle fibers that weren't being used to "pick up the slack," peaking at around 60% once fatigue is signaled.[181] It is remarkable that even when experiencing extreme, debilitating fatigue, your body may in fact have 40% of your muscle mass still available for use.

It's clear the brain is involved in making cost/benefit analyses between the effort required from muscles and the likelihood they may be damaged. Fatigue, it turns out, is closer to an emotion—an incredible system of brain and muscle interaction designed to protect the human body from harm.

There is evidence dysfunction in the hypothalamus may be the root of the problem. By blocking neuronal activity in specific nuclei within the hypothalamus, researchers reduced rats exercise performance, giving the indication that this part of the brain may be involved in the production of fatigue.[182] Just like many of the other hypersensitivities discussed in this book, it may be possible that hypothalamus dysfunction triggers off-the-scale sensitivities to the biological mechanisms that signal fatigue. As one study put it:

> *"…it would appear that CFS patients have a lower threshold for sensation during exercise compared with the normal subjects. Heightened awareness of sensations from exercising muscle due to increased afferent activity has been suggested as a possible explanation of the symptoms experienced by these patients."*[183]

In studies that compare CFS patients with controls, there would appear to be no physical differences between their skeletal muscles. If they were to use electrical stimulation to involuntarily contract their leg muscles, both groups might show equal strength, even stamina. The difference is the CFS brain might signal complete fatigue based on a trace amount of tiredness that a normal brain might ignore. To be clear, this is not a voluntary act in any way—it is a result of physiological damage to the hypothalamus.

This is only one component of the debilitating physical effects of chronic fatigue syndrome, but could explain why rest may not provide healing or restoration. The muscles were fine all along—hours or even days of sleep will not restore what wasn't exhausted. The hypothalamus is the problem—it is signaling fatigue where there is essentially none.

The effect would be exacerbated by physical exertion. If the brain can erroneously signal fatigue just from the muscular effects of lying down, it is not hard to imagine it amplifying the effects of something as simple as walking into the kitchen and pouring a glass of water into an overwhelming sensation of crippling full-body malaise. Even so, localized fatigue is still possible—the neuronal pathways are not crossed or confused, just amplified. Holding one's arm out in front of you would generate exhaustion in just that arm like any normal person, albeit at a massively accelerated rate.

A dysfunctional hypothalamus can cause tiredness in another way beyond fatigue—it can disrupt the chemicals that regulate the circadian rhythm. A proper sleep/wake cycle allows the body to get sleep at night, resting the brain, regenerating cells and restoring hormone levels. This might explain why someone who is suffering from full body fatigue can't get to sleep. After a night of sleeplessness, they may sleep through the day, only to wake up the next night, feeling just as fatigued as they were two days earlier. If you've ever traveled internationally, you will understand how horrible it would be to feel perpetual jet lag, no matter how much sleep you got.

An inflamed hypothalamus can also cause problems due to the way it overreacts to stress. There is a strange commonality amongst chronic fatigue patients you will occasionally see: childhood trauma. For many, it may be emotional distress from an overbearing parent. For others, it may be from sexual assault. Although the relationship is not clearly understood, there is an undeniable association between extreme pediatric stressors and a later onset of chronic fatigue. I believe the reason for this actually points towards the hypothalamus as a source for chronic fatigue.

In a study done on rats exposed to acute stress (in the form of restraint), the hypothalamus response was much more prolonged in prepubescent animals, leading researchers to suggest the adult hypothalamus response to stress could be profoundly shaped by pediatric events.[184] If your hypothalamus is already predisposed to a heightened stress response, dysfunction from chronic inflammation may make it even worse, triggering the release of extreme amounts of cortisol.

Cortisol is one of several hormones the body uses to prepare itself for a response to stress—it powers up your body, getting it ready for fighting or fleeing. With your body full of cortisol, it diverts all energy away from anything unnecessary for your immediate survival—this includes digestion and your immune system. A rush of cortisol may temporarily give you super-human abilities, making the difference between life and death in the wild, but it comes with a cost.

Chronically elevated cortisol levels can make you feel extremely anxious—all the time. They may be so severe they trigger frequent panic attacks, even when there is no apparent threat you can point to. You may complain to your doctor about feeling unnaturally anxious or depressed, and they may point to the fact that you are very sick and it's making you feel bad about yourself. You may instinctively know they are wrong, but are unable to point to another cause. The reality is, extremely high cortisol levels can trigger these emotions even though you have a positive attitude about your sickness and are otherwise not feeling stressed.

This scenario can also make you have trouble remembering things or concentrating, particularly noticeable by a newfound inability to do simple math problems. Elevated cortisol can also cause gastrointestinal problems. If the energy required to digest your food is reduced, you may have problems with diarrhea. If the energy required to move your food through your intestines—called gut motility—is impaired, you may end up with constipation. You may even experience both, a very painful and exhausting phenomenon. If this sounds like *irritable bowel syndrome* to you, then it probably is—you can forget about the labels—your bowel is irritable, and the symptoms listed on different websites may not line up exactly with what you are experiencing.

A final assault on your body from elevated cortisol levels is a suppressed immune system. It is a tragic irony that the chronic inflammation causing your suffering in the first place is also suppressing your immune system in such a way it's likely to never get ahead. This is why man-made diseases are so terrible—they make you very sick in ways we don't understand and can twist doctor's attempts at helping into preventing you from healing.

The effects of complete exhaustion, the inability to have restful sleep, and chronically elevated levels of cortisol may manifest in your body in the ways I've described—but also many others. If you have symptoms of extreme fatigue, your hypothalamus is probably functioning very poorly and is the cause of many of your problems. If you have a few symptoms that do not appear in the list, or are missing some that I've mentioned, read the next section on fibromyalgia and thalamus dysfunction to see if that might explain what you're experiencing.

FIBROMYALGIA

Sitting just behind and above the hypothalamus is another important component of the brain called the thalamus. The thalamus is unique in that every sensory system in your body (besides smell) has a special nucleus in this part of your brain. And even though your olfactory system does not have a nucleus in the thalamus, it still runs through there.

The same mechanisms that I described with hypothalamus might apply with fibromyalgia. Portions of your thalamus may be damaged by metals arriving via white blood cells, but the long-term suffering associated with fibromyalgia may be additionally due to chronic inflammation from an intracellular bacterial infection—an infection your body cannot rid itself of.

We have seen earlier in the book how problems with motor nerves tend to cause weakness and problems with sensory nerves tend to cause hypersensitivity. The thalamus is the mothership of sensory management in your body, and if it's not functioning properly, you may experience hypersensitivity in every single aspect of your life.

The smell of ink on a newspaper may make you faint. A whispered conversation from down the hall may prevent you from working. The sounds of crowds or washing dishes can give you headaches. The screen on your phone could feel like blinding light. The ability to sense and regulate temperature in different parts of your body can be impaired. The motion sickness from a simple car ride can become unbearable.[i]

Scientific studies have shown that with an impaired thalamus, decision making can become very difficult.[185] It can affect your ability to concentrate and keep your train of thought while you are talking. It can even affect your sense of consciousness, a phenomenon that many fibromyalgia sufferers refer to as "brain fog." If you have experienced this effect, you will know that is a very particular sensation that's different than what you might experience if sleep-deprived. It's been described as being awake and aware, but with an unnerving ability to get your brain to do what you want.

The worst part is the pain—burning, unbearable pain in nearly any part of your body. The thalamus is largely responsible for modulating the perception of pain in your body everywhere.[186] If it's dysfunctional, it can make the slightest touch feel like a rusty kitchen knife. Your skin can feel like 3rd or 4th degree sunburn, your joints like balls of sand spurs. The inside your body isn't safe either, as the sensory nerves from muscles and even organs can create sharp, localized stabbing pains—or a dull, full-body ache that makes even lying down uncomfortable.

For someone who has never experienced these symptoms, it can sound so surreal that it defies belief. How could anyone live through that kind of pain, you might ask. I have been so moved by the people who heroically endure this illness, often without the support of their family and friends. They press on, every day, in an attempt to reclaim

---

i. If you have a constellation of several sensory issues—like smell and sound and light, it's likely caused by dysfunction with your thalamus. If you have a single sensory issue, like a vestibulocochlear dysfunction, it's probably a cranial nerve palsy due to acute metal toxicity.

their health and gain their lives back.

As your body wages an epic battle against the infection in your brain, the symptoms might oscillate between fibromyalgia and chronic fatigue syndrome. You may have started your journey with a crystal clear chronic fatigue diagnosis only to have it shift into the debilitating pain of fibromyalgia years later.

What happens if the infection moves beyond this specific area of the brain? You will start to see other "diseases" appear on your medical chart. Lupus and rheumatoid arthritis are commonly associated with these conditions. We know that fibromyalgia creates joint pain, but without the visible swelling of rheumatoid arthritis or lupus. If the bacterial infection causing fibromyalgia or CFS moves into a more aggressive phase—or perhaps a new infection is picked up—it can trigger the acute inflammation associated with those diseases. As your body's white blood cells become depleted from intracellular bacteria, additional "co-infections" become easier and easier to acquire.

Fibromyalgia patients sometimes speak of going out in the sun and developing skin rashes, something they attribute to their temperature sensitivity when in fact, it is a diagnostic criterion for lupus. Sjögren's syndrome and thyroid problems can also appear, only to go away months later. Even some of the Ehler-Danlos syndromes, currently a group of 13 connective tissue disorders[ii], commonly share symptoms from fibromyalgia and CFS. And they can all exhibit traits of postural orthostatic tachycardia syndrome (POTS)—the illness that can make standing or even sitting cause fainting or unconsciousness.

The good news is if the theories put forth in this book are correct, healing and recovery should be possible from these diseases. Their completely debilitating effects could simply be the result of chronic

---

ii. Ehler-Danlos clearly demonstrates the difficulties in diagnosing modern-disease—there are infinite variations.

inflammation in a specific area of your brain, and indeed, there are many who have had complete recoveries from fibromyalgia and chronic fatigue syndrome by addressing long-running infections. Based on the success of others, and until science proves otherwise, I would assume that a complete recovery is possible.

CHRONIC LYME DISEASE

Chronic Lyme disease is another tricky attempt at labeling that causes confusion. Lyme disease, without the "chronic" label, refers to the effects of a *Borrelia burgdorferi* infection—a specific illness associated with a tick bite. "Chronic" Lyme disease originally referred to a grouping of symptoms that were attributed to the lingering effects of a Lyme infection.

Long after the initial tick-bite infection had cleared, people would begin to complain of debilitating fatigue, muscle aches, brain fog or joint pains. It seemed that something was causing this once short-term illness to become a chronic infection. Over time, people became aware of these symptoms, and those that experienced similar effects thought they might also be experiencing the after-effects of a Lyme infection—despite not having suffered from the original illness or a tick bite.

These people were sometimes diagnosed with chronic Lyme and as more people began to experience these symptoms, awareness of the disease grew. At the same time, other people began to experience similar symptoms but lived in areas where ticks did not. Some people with these symptoms lived in tick borne areas but were positive they had never been bitten by a tick. These people could not have chronic Lyme and would end up with other diagnoses like chronic fatigue syndrome or fibromyalgia.

Whereas chronic fatigue syndrome and fibromyalgia are not associated with a particular pathogen, chronic Lyme disease is. People do not challenge chronic fatigue or fibromyalgia diagnoses because there is no blood test to question it with. Chronic Lyme is essentially the same set of symptoms but associated with specific bacteria—a bacteria for which a test *does* exist.

One problem—depending on the stage of the disease, the test may show a negative result even though there is an active infection going on. Additionally, the test cannot confirm the presence of the bacteria, but only the presence of antibodies to the bacteria. It shows that at some point in your life, the bacteria were present in your body and your immune system generated a response to it.[i]

In short, the test may be negative when it should be positive, and even a positive result doesn't mean much. Many people have had a Borrelia burgdorferi infection at some point in their life and have no chronic symptoms to show for it. Others show all the symptoms of chronic Lyme disease but have negative test results for the Lyme bacteria.

Because of all of this, many very sick people have ended up feeling like the existence of their illness was being questioned. If they would have lived in California and received a chronic fatigue or fibromyalgia diagnosis, they might not have had a problem—their diagnosis would not have been met with skepticism. Also, bacterial infections are not often suspected with chronic fatigue and fibromyalgia, even though they may have the exact same symptoms. Consequently, their

---

i. There are more sophisticated tests but are not affordable or readily available to the public.

treatment regimens would have differed. Chronic Lyme *is* associated with particular bacteria, and as such, is often treated aggressively (and erroneously we will find) with antibiotics.

All of these disorders may be due to the same thing—chronic inflammation caused by long-running bacterial infections. None of them would happen without the presence of metals or massive antibiotics in the body. Like Zika and CTE, it is not the virus or the head trauma, but the combination of these things along with metal that has turned a once fairly innocuous infection into the possibility of a crippling illness.

Zika has existed in countries for hundreds of years without causing birth defects until recently. Men have been smashing their heads against each other for thousands of years with little long-lasting neurodegenerative effects until recently. People have been getting bitten by ticks with little more than an acute, short-term illness for thousands of years until recently.

These once trivial events have been transformed into something far more sinister ever since metals or antibiotics were introduced into the body. Although metals may be giving the bacteria that ticks introduce into the body the intracellular boost they need to create very nasty infections, the antibiotics may be doing just as much harm.

If you get a tick bite, you should assume you are infected with Lyme and immediately start an antibiotic. Ignore what you might read about the bulls-eye rash—it's meaningless. The test is meaningless, especially in these early stages. You may get a false positive which will convince your doctor you don't need antibiotics. Antibiotics are the first line of treatment against Lyme disease and often work well if you treat it right away.

However, if you wait until much later, or as is the case with most people, if you had no idea you were even carrying the bacteria, the antibiotics are likely to make the infection worse. They may work for a little while and will make you feel slightly better. They are killing some of the bacteria, but the main reason you feel better initially is because the spirochetes are going into hiding.

Spirochetes are very nasty critters and besides the intracellular problem common with other bacterial infections discussed in this book, they have a couple of their own tricks. If they sense they are under attack from antibiotics, they may burrow into tissue to escape. Their very shape allows them to spiral into places that normal bacteria could never get—even past the blood brain barrier—a possible factor in the chronic inflammation seen in Alzheimer's.

Spirochetes can also curl up into a ball and form a cyst around themselves. If the antibiotics are administered early, before the bacteria has had a chance to proliferate, it can kill enough of them that your body's immune system can get ahead of the infection. If it is later, during a more active infection, there may be enough of them that they can hide and wait it out until you stop administering antibiotics.

Once you stop the antibiotics, the cysts sense that it's safe and can release multiple versions of themselves as they change back into their original form, exponentially increasing their numbers. When this happens, you will feel suddenly worse than ever and most likely will go back on the antibiotics in a never-ending cycle.

Chronic fatigue and fibromyalgia are just variations of chronic Lyme disease. They may have the same bacteria or perhaps different ones. They may even have combinations of ones that overlap, but we really have no way of knowing. The unfortunate reality is unless you were to do a biopsy on the thalamus and hypothalamus in your brain and check for specific bacterial infection, it will be very hard to determine the microbial source of inflammation. It feels like science or medicine should be further along than this, but these sorts of tests are very difficult to do on living human beings.

It would be foolish to suppose you could not pick up a Borrelia burgdorferi infection from anywhere other than tick bites. It would also be foolish to suppose that many other bacterial infections could not cause the exact same inflammation as the Lyme spirochete. Many people currently diagnosed with chronic Lyme disease may have never had a Borrelia burgdorferi infection at all. Others diagnosed with chronic Lyme may test positive for Lyme but are in fact dealing with an infection from different bacteria. And lastly, many people with chronic fatigue or fibromyalgia may actually be dealing with the long-term effects of a raging Lyme infection but have never been tested for it.

As I mentioned in the beginning of the chapter, chronic Lyme clearly illustrates the limitations of labeling clusters of symptoms in the same way we think of classical microbial or genetic disease. It is my hope that as medicine moves forward in its understanding of how man-made diseases are formed and sustained, we can learn to classify them in such a way that promotes healing rather than preventing it.

RHEUMATOID ARTHRITIS

Rheumatoid arthritis (RA), juvenile rheumatoid arthritis (JRA) and juvenile idiopathic arthritis (JVI) are similar to chronic fatigue syndrome, fibromyalgia and chronic Lyme. They are vague diagnoses that sometimes fit and sometimes don't. You might think you are the textbook definition of RA, but wait a few months and either you or the text book will change. Probably both.

A quick read through the symptoms of RA lists many things beyond joint pain and inflammation that involve other organs and wildly varying symptoms like dry eyes and mouth, scarring in the lungs, even fatigue and tiredness. It's no wonder doctors have such a difficult time diagnosing illness these days—the hundreds of disorders and conditions overlap each other in multiple ways.

The cause of RA may be the same for many of these other diseases: either metal toxicity or chronic intracellular bacterial inflammation enabled by metal and/or antibiotics. If you have fatigue or tiredness, your hypothalamus is probably being damaged in the same way as chronic fatigue patients. Nodules under the skin and scarring in the eyes or lungs is indicative of granulomatous issues covered in the lupus and sarcoidosis chapter. Regardless, all of these problems are just other symptoms of the same thing. You may have one or multiple bacterial infections causing them and though the medical treatment may differ between them, the cure will be the same.

Let's focus on the common symptom of RA—joint pain. Even this hallmark symptom is inconsistent amongst patients—some have swelling, others have no swelling. Some have markers in their blood for inflammation, others have none. Steroids help some people, others not. Descriptions of the disease often conflict themselves:

> *"Inflammation causes redness, swelling, warmth, and soreness in the joints, although many children with JRA do not complain of joint pain…"*[187]

You can imagine why parents might throw their hands in the air. When patients are screaming of joint pain and a thorough examination of problem areas (including X-rays) doesn't reveal a single indication of inflammation, you can imagine why doctors would be frustrated.

With no visible sign of inflammation, a physician may order a test to prove you are not crazy. The C-reactive protein (CRP) test looks for a marker of inflammation in the body—anywhere in the body. Most people experiencing any of the non-joint issues I've described above are likely to show inflammation. With no visible inflammation in your joints and a CRP test that indicated inflammation, the puzzle becomes even more confusing.

Your physician may then order a rheumatoid factor test. This test is actually thought to be indicative of autoimmune activity in many other diseases such as lupus, sarcoidosis, Sjögren's and leukemia. Rheumatoid factor is a name for what they call an *autoantibody*. An autoantibody is an antibody that for reasons unknown appears to attack your own tissues. This concept forms the basis of autoimmune theory but is very poorly understood. For instance, it is thought your body may purposefully develop autoantibodies to help it kill cancer cells.

Because of this, a positive rheumatoid factor test can be interpreted as something going wrong but perhaps it indicates that something is actually going right—your body has sensed a stealthy invader and is doing everything it can to get rid of it. If your body were to take action against white blood cells full of aluminum or intracellular bacteria, you could understand why—to an outside observer who could spot neither aluminum or intracellular bacteria—your immune system might appear to be perplexed. Although molecular mimicry surely does occur, I believe the "confusion" displayed by your immune system is actually a purposeful, coordinated attempt to kill white blood cells full of aluminum or intracellular bacteria in your body. If this is what's happening, it may be the true foundation of autoimmunity—a foundation which might easily be undone.

If you can put the diagnoses and labels aside for a few moments and focus on joint pain, I believe you can split it down the middle into two distinct categories: joint pain with localized swelling and/or inflammation and joint pain without any apparent swelling or inflammation. The reason for this difference is fascinating.

If you are experiencing joint pain and can easily detect swelling and inflammation, there may be a fairly simple diagnosis: bacterial infection. The chronic inflammation caused by these microbes will trigger visible signs of tissue injury easily spotted by your physician. Your body may not be able to clear these bacteria because they have become intracellular versions of their original selves, or your immune system may be so suppressed due to chronic infections going on elsewhere that it is unable to clear the infection.

Studies have associated many different types of bacterial infections with RA, notably the microbes which cause periodontal disease and urinary tract infections.[188] Could the tooth eruption of childhood provide frequent opportunities for *P. gingivalis* and other bacteria to gain entry into the bloodstream? There are many different bacteria associated with joint pain and it seems these bacteria have a special affinity for synovial joints throughout your body, often thriving there to cause tremendous pain. In a properly functioning immune system, your body should be able to clear these bacterial infections easily. If the bacteria have become intracellular and are replicating within white blood cells, it becomes much more difficult and these infections can get out of control.

As environmental factors change around you, such as stress from moving to a new city or the immune activation changes from pregnancy, you will feel your symptoms wax and wane as your body gets ahead or behind the infection. You may have a complete relapse due to a stretch of good luck—a new relationship that brings you joy. A promotion at work. Dietary changes that introduce probiotics into your intestines and give your immune system a break from all the resources it had been devoting to your gut. Any of these things may supercharge your immune system in such a way it is able to get on top of these chronic infections. But due to the metal in your body, the occasional use of antibiotics, a reintroduction of stress, or many other environmental factors, your immune system may begin to lose the battle against these bacteria and your symptoms will return.

If you have visibly inflamed joints alongside other issues like swollen lymph nodes or irritated eyes, you are likely fighting a chronic bacterial infection throughout your body—a battle which your immune system is losing. Because our understanding of the interaction between antibiotics and intracellular bacteria is incomplete, you might take an antibiotic that actually makes you worse. Take a look through the Healing and Recovery chapter of this book for some quick ideas on how to get rid of these infections.

* * *

The first type of joint pain can be ascribed to physical inflammation from bacterial infections and are visible to both the naked eye and X-rays. The other joint pain—no physical inflammation—is the kind that can cause patients and doctors to lose their minds.

As researchers have tried to pinpoint the nature of how these microbes may be causing rheumatoid arthritis, they've been consistently flummoxed by one thing—many people show no signs of inflammation. It as if their joints are completely fine. Similar to the muscles in patients with chronic fatigue, they may be perfect specimens of anatomical health. What is going on with these people?

Within the joints between your bones lie four different types of nerve endings. These sensors each have unique functions but all work together in order to: 1) relay positional information to your brain about where your body is in space, and 2) prevent you from injuring your joints by stretching them too far. In a design that industrial robots have copied, your brain not only commands your muscles to move to a particular location, it interprets information from sensors within the connective tissue of the joints and can detect and confirm those movements.

These sensors are present in all of your joints and run through the nervous system into your brain, terminating in the thalamus. If you haven't read the chapter on fibromyalgia, the thalamus is the sensory processing center of your brain. Nearly everything that requires input from sensory information around your body passes through here. Lesions on your brain from metal toxicity or inflammation from long running infections can cause your thalamus to work incorrectly—a phenomenon which has been shown to cause terrible pain in parts of your body.[189][i]

If you develop a problem in a very specific part of the thalamus,

---

i. Look up *vasculitis* for more specific information as to how inflammation can damage the thalamus.

you can begin to experience extreme pain in your neck or shoulders. Another area might cause your skin to feel like it's on fire. In both cases, there is nothing wrong with those tissues, but the communication system supposed to detect and relay actual pain. Similarly, a lesion or inflammation in a slightly different area of the thalamus might cause crippling joint pain as it misinterprets the signals coming in from all of the nerve sensors in the synovial joints around your body.

The pain could come and go and even move around to various parts of your body as the neurons in your damaged thalamus try to repair themselves. The pain might be worse as you move, as the dysfunctioning thalamus could be amplifying any signal it receives one thousand times over. In the same way that fibromyalgia patients feel excruciating pain in various parts of their body, you may have a subset of that pain—specific to the joints. For some reason, people can accept that areas like your face or skin may occasionally experience pain but have a very difficult time accepting this same concept could also happen to a collection of nerves grouped more by function than location.

If you have joint pain with no visible swelling or signs of inflammation, you and your doctor will likely have questioned your sanity along the way. Hopefully, it may bring you some peace knowing that something as simple as dysfunction within the thalamus could explain exactly what you're feeling. Two other things may point towards the thalamus as the source of your troubles—if you experience joint pains and they move in perfect symmetry around your body, that also may indicate a neurological origin. Microbial infections are not likely to progress in that way—not impossible, but unlikely.

Secondly, if you also experience fatigue or tiredness alongside your joint pains, it might indicate a problem in that area of your brain, as the thalamus also plays a part in your sleep and wakefulness.[190] Finally, you may have a combination of both of these scenarios. You may have symmetrical joint pain caused by thalamic inflammation but also have a particular spot on one side of your body with true, visible inflammation. Both of these issues might be due to the same microbe causing an infection in your brain and in the joints themselves.

For those of you who have dealt with the horrors of rheumatoid arthritis for years, this theory may come as a shock. Although both causes of joint pain I've described in this chapter are vastly different, they are likely to be caused by the same thing. This common origin might lead to a cluster of overlapping symptoms that will perplex the most astute patient—RA with visible inflammation and RA without a sign of inflammation. If you have been confounded by the lack of a plausible explanation for why you have been suffering, I hope this hypothesis provides a crack in the door towards healing.

TYPE 1 DIABETES

Jane and her family were staying in a hotel when one of her children got sick. It was a stomach bug, and in the closed quarters of a tiny hotel room, they all got it, making what would have been a nice trip miserable. Within two weeks, they were back at home and everyone had recovered from the bug. Her oldest son, 11, was showing some new symptoms of something she had never seen before.

"He started drinking a lot," she said, "like way more than normal, to the point he wasn't sleeping well at night because he had to get up so often to use the bathroom. He couldn't seem to make it in a five-minute car ride without needing to stop."

Her son's condition would continue to deteriorate over the next few days until she decided to measure his blood sugar with a meter she happened to have at the house.

"I took his blood sugar and it was 753. Called the doctor and left for the Children's Hospital ER."

It was *type 1 diabetes*. His pancreas had stopped working and it could've killed him. He had gone from a perfectly healthy eleven-year old to needing insulin shots to keep him alive in under four weeks.

Type 2 diabetes, the more common kind of diabetes, occurs when the body is unable to process insulin correctly. This condition is most often attributed to genetics and lifestyle choices. Many people who are suffering from this type of diabetes can reverse its effects through dietary and exercise modifications. It's mentioned frequently throughout history and appears to have existed for a very long time.

Type 1 diabetes appears to be a relatively recent phenomenon. It was previously known as *juvenile diabetes* because of its tendency to occur in children, but that characteristic is quickly disappearing. The mechanism which causes issues in type 1 is different than its more prevalent sibling. In this kind of diabetes, the pancreas develops a problem and cannot produce enough insulin. It's thought to be an autoimmune disorder where the body begins to attack the *beta cells* in the pancreas—cells responsible for creating and storing insulin.

As Jane began to reach out to other mothers with children who had suddenly developed type 1 diabetes, she noticed a pattern.

"Stomach bugs," she said. "It was so common. Perfectly healthy child, no history of any serious illness, gets a stomach bug and a few weeks later they're diagnosed. I even met a lady with siblings that had both gotten a bug and both developed diabetes within a few weeks. It's crazy."

Because identical twins rarely both get type 1, it is assumed that environmental factors play a large part in its onset.[191] Another woman wrote me with the account of her diagnosis.

"I was diagnosed at age 22. The last thing before I was diagnosed was a lingering, month-long wet cough followed by a course of antibiotics."

A study I found looked at the impact of orally-administered aluminum on pancreatic beta cells in rats but found them to be unchanged.[192] There are many different studies looking at the impact of aluminum on a particular area of the body, but because of what we now know about aluminum translocation, this type of research is unlikely to reveal what we would like. These studies often administer the aluminum orally, which severely limits the uptake of the metal into the body. Secondly, they operate on the assumption that absorbed aluminum dissipates evenly into the body, when we now believe that aluminum doesn't disperse randomly but is signaled to specific locations based on immune activation.

Could these infections be the trigger that causes aluminum to rush into the pancreas and destroy the beta cells responsible for insulin production? For our concerns, a more telling study might inject aluminum into the rats, then expose them to a virus, such as the norovirus, and check their pancreatic function.

Both rotavirus and the rotavirus vaccine have been linked to the onset of type 1 diabetes, ostensibly because the virus has a similarity to a component of the pancreas.[193] It is thought this might trigger autoimmunity by molecular mimicry. It's also clear that viruses can directly affect the pancreas as the Influenza A virus can cause pancreatitis in animal models, leading to a form of diabetes.[194]

Reading through the literature on the role infections might play in diabetes, I noticed that work-related exposure to aluminum and cadmium—another type of metal—caused a significant increase in *pancreatic cancer*.[195] Because rates for this horrible disease are on the rise, I'd be curious if its onset could be traced back to an infection that inadvertently signaled metal that had been stored around the body towards it. Because the progression of pancreatic cancer is slow, pointing towards a particular trigger will be difficult, but obviously the concept of specific infections drawing metals into particular organs could explain much.

Something is causing type 1 diabetes—it is not purely a genetic predisposition. There is a significant environmental factor at play, and I believe it may be a viral infection and aluminum doing the damage.

I will close with a prophetic, ominous realization from Etienne Lanceraux, the Frenchman who in the 1880s did much to advance the early understanding of diabetes:

> 'A disease', as he pointed out, 'corresponds to a special cause, to a particular course, to constant anatomical lesions. But nothing like this exists for diabetes mellitus: its cause is unknown, its course so variable, that some patients could live 40 years and more, while others die after only 2 or 3 years.'[196]

The era of bacteria and viruses had gotten more complicated. Disease, it would seem, was on the way out. But a thousand new disorders, syndromes and spectrums—with courses variable and causes unknown—were ready to take their place.

SARCOIDOSIS

Sarcoidosis starts for many as a few spots on their face. They may be subtle discoloration or obvious and painful. A frustrating visit to the dermatologist may yield no answers and then after a few months, the patient might begin to notice a persistent cough, even though they don't feel sick.

In sarcoidosis, the white blood cells can form granulomas in places where there's no apparent infection going on. This often happens in the lungs, where it can cause coughing, shortness of breath or chest pain, but can also happen in the lymph nodes, the gallbladder, the bones, joints, nerves, even the skin or eyes. Besides being painful, sarcoidosis granulomas can be mistaken for lung cancer, an error that's not comforting when lymph node granulomas have been associated with non-Hodgkin's lymphoma, a type of cancer.[197]

A common symptom of sarcoidosis is called *erythema nodosum*— tender red nodules under the skin. Interestingly, this same effect can be seen in rheumatoid arthritis, lupus, and strep throat infections. The fact that even a strep infection can cause these same nodules gives indication there is a microbial component to sarcoidosis.

There is one bacteria that consistently comes up in sarcoidosis—*Propionibacterium acnes*. P. acnes has consistently been found in sarcoid lymph nodes and granulomas, but has also been cultured in patients *without* sarcoidosis—found in 24 of 43 lungs[198] and 10 of 20 gastric lymph nodes. The bacteria associated with sarcoidosis appears to be prevalent in many people who don't exhibit any granulomas. Why might some people with the disease have problems when others don't?

As researchers began picking apart the sarcoid granulomas, they found what appeared to be intracellular forms of P. acnes bacteria. This is concerning because these same types of bacteria have also been associated with appendicitis, cirrhosis, lymphoid tumors, colon carcinoma, and many other[199] illnesses.

The difference appears to be attributable to the form of the bacteria. If you remember back to the chapter on Crohn's disease, experiments with *Streptococcus faecalis* bacteria failed to create granulomatous inflammation in the intestines of rabbits. When the exact same bacteria were introduced *without their cell wall*—granulomas formed, just like in humans. Crohn's disease is called a granulomatous disease because inflammation in the intestines form granulomas—just like we see in sarcoidosis. With sarcoidosis, granulomas form in a variety of places—usually starting in the lymph nodes of the lungs.

If you think back to the Crohn's disease chapter once more, you will remember the reason inflammation normally starts in that particular area of the small intestine is because of a special type of lymphoid tissue called Peyer's patches that surround the terminal ileum. Like any other lymph tissue, Peyer's patches collect aluminum-containing white blood cells and give any bacteria nearby plenty of opportunity to change into their intracellular form. From this location, the inflammation from various intracellular bacteria cause granulomas to form along the intestinal walls as the infection proliferates.

Peyer's patches aren't the only specialized lymphoid tissues—they are also present in several other areas throughout your body. One of these other places is within the lungs and perhaps not by coincidence, the granulomas associated with sarcoidosis often start in the lungs.

The P. acnes bacteria present in many people may cause an infection and immune response with little fanfare. For those who have a significant accumulation of aluminum in the lymphoid tissue in their lungs, they make take a turn for the worse as the metal transforms the bacteria into its intracellular form, allowing it to proliferate in the white blood cells, avoid detection and wreck the immune system in the process.

Many people won't notice an issue in their lungs until much later in the infection when their cough has become persistent enough they have it X-rayed. Unlike the intestines, where 70% of your immune system exists to prevent invaders from getting into your body, the blood and lymphatic systems that perfuse your lungs offer no such protection. With Crohn's, the infection is typically contained to areas near the site of the initial infection. When this same sequence of events happens in the lymphatic system around your lungs, the lymphatic and blood systems may carry the out of control infection anywhere—your gall bladder, your face, your eyes and certainly other lymph nodes around your body.

It is fascinating that an illness as seemingly unalike as Crohn's might serve as a nearly perfect model for the way in which sarcoidosis begins and sustains its destruction. The concept of an initial surge of intracellular bacteria due to an accumulation of aluminum in specialized lymphoid tissue around the body may also be the origin of other illnesses such as thyroid disorders and breast cancer.

SYSTEMIC LUPUS ERYTHEMATOSUS

Diseases of the skin have come and gone throughout medical literature. In the 1850s, something different began to appear. Not only was the characteristic butterfly rash visible on people's faces, but it appeared to move around the body, even causing joint pain and damage to internal organs. Another concerning feature of the new disease—its symptoms could disappear, only to return years later. At that time, surviving an infection was known to provide a lifetime of immunity. This illness, like some of the other strange disorders that began to appear around then could come and go multiple times.

The disorder was named *systemic lupus erythematosus* (SLE).[i] "Systemic" was added to the previous label to indicate the all-encompassing nature of the new illness. New symptoms like joint pain, chest pain, and fatigue accompanied this once simple illness—even confusion and memory loss are sometimes associated with it. What might be causing this terrible illness? Genetic predisposition appears to

---

i. This book refers to SLE as lupus for simplicity's sake.

have very little to do with whether you get lupus or not. If someone with an identical twin gets lupus, the other twin has only a 25% chance of also getting it—a statistic that would indicate mostly environmental causes.

A breakthrough in lupus research came out of the Mayo Clinic lab in 1948. Scientists discovered a new type of "entity" in the bone marrow of patients with lupus—a special type of cell that was difficult for them to identify. After refining their technique, they realized this new cell could also be found in the blood of lupus patients but in numbers usually too few to spot.

They named it the lupus erythematosus cell (LE cell) because it only seemed to be present in patients with lupus. Since then, detection techniques have improved and LE cells can be found in lupus patients within the fluid around their joints, their spine, their heart, and their lungs. The cell is so unique to lupus, it can be used to test for the disorder.

What was so distinctive about the LE Cell? It exhibited a trait they had never seen before—it was a type of white blood cell that contained the nucleus of another cell inside it. LE cells, were simply white blood cells with intracellular bacteria inside. They may not have been able to see the intracellular bacteria, but once inside the white blood cells, the abnormalities they created were easily visible.

We have seen how a couple of disorders like Crohn's disease and sarcoidosis may get their start in special lymphoid tissues around the body. In Crohn's disease, it's the Peyer's patches in the terminal ileum. With sarcoidosis, it's the bronchial-associated lymphoid tissue within the lungs. The frequent shape and location of the butterfly rash seen wrapping around the cheeks of many with lupus may initiate from metal and intracellular bacteria infecting the *maxillary sinus* or the *nasolabial lymph node*.

This tissue may accumulate aluminum just like other lymphoid tissues and give rise to an intracellular form of bacteria—LE cells – that start within the facial tissue and move throughout the body. While specific bacteria aren't frequently associated with lupus, we can assume that whatever they are gain their intracellular form due to metals gathered in lymphoid tissue around the body. Most bacteria have a preference for particular areas, and the bacteria inside LE cells seem to have a preference for the blood vessels that line the skin, joints and membranes around the lungs and heart.

When their numbers are high enough, they can cause inflammation in the blood vessels, swelling them to such an extent that blood begins to leak into the surrounding tissue—an event that causes the redness you see in many of the different lupus-related rashes.[ii] If the skin gets hot, blood vessels naturally dilate in an attempt to release heat from the body. This is designed to create sweat, something which will cool someone down as it evaporates. In a lupus patient, where blood vessels are already inflamed, the reaction to the heat from sun-exposure can often be enough additional dilation to leak blood into surrounding tissue, causing what some call "sun poisoning."

If the infection continues unchecked, enough LE cells may gather in the joints that their inflammation causes painful swelling. More LE cells can pool in the membranes around the lungs, causing it to hurt when you inhale. Even the membranes in your brain can become inflamed in a similar way, leading to headaches and confusion.

As the LE cells proliferate throughout the body, the immune system becomes increasingly ineffective. The bacteria are replicating inside white blood cells and are not being tagged for destruction by your immune system. As more and more of your white-blood cells are inhabited by these bacteria, the effectiveness of your immune system

---

ii. Occasionally, the LE cells can cause blood vessels to contract, leading to poor blood circulation in those areas and the white and blue fingers that comes with that.

goes down. If you were to get extremely stressed or sick with the flu or a cold in this depressed state, the effects might become much worse.

As I have mentioned with the other disorders, if these theories about what is causing lupus are correct, then healing from this horrible illness should theoretically be possible. It is simply a chronic bacterial infection that your immune system is having a very difficult time overcoming. While there are metals and/or certain antibiotics in your body causing intracellular forms of this bacteria to form, you will have a very difficult time controlling this infection. You may temporarily beat the infection, possibly even for years, but the next time you encounter the bacteria, or possibly from the immune suppression that comes from extreme stress or pregnancy, it may come raging back worse than before.

Read the chapter on healing and recovery for ideas about how to get started recovering from the chronic infections that may be causing lupus.

THE PROBLEM WITH VITAMIN D

Think about this confusing state of affairs: our foods are fortified with vitamin D, we're getting too much sun exposure, and our bodies can produce as much as 20,000 IUs in just thirty minutes. But according to some scientists, vitamin D deficiency is growing?[200] Another study found vitamin D deficiencies in Israel—a very sunny country in which one would not expect to find such a problem.[201] These statements ought to leave you scratching your head.

Vitamin D is actually not a vitamin at all but a *secosteroid hormone*. We can't make vitamin D on our own but get it from exposure to sunlight, multivitamins, fish, eggs, or milk and cereal where it is artificially added.

In a healthy individual with a robust immune system, vitamin D isn't normally an issue. Within their kidneys, the native form—*25,D*—is converted into the active form—*1,25 D*—and levels are regulated to match the body's needs. Under normal circumstances, vitamin D boosts the immune system and helps the body create its own "natural antibiotics"—called *antimicrobial peptides*—that are designed to kill off pathogens. In those with a compromised immune system who have chronic illness caused by metals and intracellular bacteria, vitamin D takes on a different role—it becomes an immune suppressor.

Many people with chronic infections are told by their doctor their lab test indicates they are deficient in vitamin D. It is easy to assume a "deficiency" may be caused by simply not getting enough, but this is not always the case. In this scenario, a low 25,D value is not the cause of their illness, and taking more will certainly not cure it.[i]

White blood cells (specifically macrophages) infected with intracellular bacteria convert 25,D to 1,25 D independent of the kidneys and can cause levels to rise far above what the body requires. This creates at least two potential problems: 1) Elevated 1,25 D increases unproductive inflammation, and 2) Intracellular bacteria produce *ligands* that bind up the Vitamin D receptors. With these receptors blocked, they can no longer effectively signal the production of antimicrobial peptides, the body's own antibiotics.

This allows bacteria to easily move in and out of the white blood cells and multiply—all just beyond the reach of the immune system. Not only are the white blood cells hijacked and unable to do their job, it also provides the opportunity for other infections like viruses, fungi, and parasites to proliferate and thrive.

Often, people are searching for the cause of their digestive problems and will say, "I think it's leaky gut, I think it's food allergies, I think it's *candida*, I think it's parasites…"

While it could be any—or all—of these things, it's important to take a step back and evaluate what might have damaged the body so badly to make it incapable of regulating any of these conditions.

Many people with a chronic disease will feel alleviation of their

---

i. You can confirm whether or not this disease process is taking place in your body by testing for both vitamin D values. Ask your doctor for a lab test to check 25, D as well as 1,25 D. A normal ratio is 1:1.1. A highly elevated 1,25 level in comparison to the 25, D will confirm intracellular bacteria causing out of control conversion from 25,D to 1,25 D. It is very important to have your specimen frozen for a more accurate result.

symptoms in the summer time when they get more sun exposure. These same people often dread the winter, as their vitamin D levels drop to an annual low—a time when they feel their symptoms most acutely. In the summer, more vitamin D will mean more 1,25 D, which will create more immunosuppression and less symptoms – an end result similar to the effects of steroids like prednisone. Similarly, less vitamin D will produce less 1,25 D, which will create less immunosuppression and more dramatic symptoms.

It's natural to prefer alleviation of symptoms. Unfortunately, this is unlikely to do anything to help the immune system address the root cause of your illness. Consuming additional vitamin D or getting extra sun to mitigate the symptoms will decrease the immune response, but has the decidedly negative side effect of helping intracellular bacteria proliferate. It's the same as using biologic pharmaceuticals like Humira or Enbrel—these medicines shut down the immune response to decrease inflammation, but not without serious consequences. They are so effective at disabling the immune system you must test negative for tuberculosis before starting them.

Autoimmune patients may hear their doctor mention that the cause of their disease is inflammation. While this may be true, it's necessary to move one step further towards actual healing and ask, "What is causing the inflammation?" The answer to that question is what you should be treating, above all.

Even though suppressing inflammation is ineffective at addressing the underlying issues of your illness, too much inflammation can also be detrimental. For example, tissue damage to your heart from severe inflammation is probably never a good thing. Purposefully lowering your vitamin D too much might produce an excessive immune response, but raising it might prevent your immune system from ever being able to heal. Striking the right balance is important.

Ideally, you should decrease inflammation enough to protect vital tissue and organs from damage, but not so much that it shuts down your immune system completely—you need your body to generate a robust immune response if it is going to be able to overcome the intracellular infections that are the cause of your illness.

This can be a difficult subject to understand. It's mentioned in the healing and recovery chapter, but for guidance on how you and your doctor can treat intracellular infections and reduce your inflammation —without suppressing your immune system—visit chronicillnessrecovery.org.

WHY YOU CAN'T TAN ANYMORE

An interesting phenomenon may help us understand the dysfunction that is happening within the body—just under the surface, actually. The variation of skin tone in humans seems to be infinite and yet, there are colorings that would seem to instinctively tell us someone is sick. Whether it's a change in tone or a particular hue that our brain locks on to, there may be an innate ability to sense illness in someone purely by reading their skin.

I had heard of this phenomenon from my wife, who showed me pictures of her at the beach as a child—a golden bronze wonder with nary a drop of sunscreen in sight. Although her coloring is a bit different now, I wouldn't have thought such a distinct change was possible until she spent several weeks one summer trying to tan. While her college friends turned a nice golden brown, they were all amazed at how it seemed the sun was going right through her—as if she had spent the entire day inside and remained a very pale shade.

It wasn't until other people began to reach out to me with their stories of similarly dramatic changes in skin coloring that I began to realize something specific was happening. A woman wrote an account of her transformation that sounded like many others I heard:

> *"As a child I always tanned very easily… spent summers at a local swimming pool. At around age 12 or 13, I went swimming and burned badly from head to toe—had never burned before. After then, I didn't tan well and tended to burn easier. As an adult I now burn just 'thinking about sun' and actually develop PLE[i] on chest, arms and face if I am in the sun for more than a few minutes. I am fairer now as an adult than I was as a child. I do not tan at all. My eye color has changed, also. I used to have brown eyes (hazel, but so much brown that anyone would have considered them as such). I now have green eyes… very little to no brown… even some blue in there—you would never think my eyes used to be brown."*

There are three different types of *melanin*, a natural pigment produced in the human body. The first two are *eumelanin* and *pheomelanin*—combinations of these pigments are what give us our different colors. Without these two pigments, everything would be white—except your skin, which would be tinted pink due to the red blood cells running just underneath its surface.

Pheomelanin is less common and is mainly responsible for anything red—like your hair. Eumelanin, the other pigment, comes in two flavors—brown and black. If you have a tiny bit of the brown eumelanin, you will have blonde hair. If you have a tiny bit of black eumelanin, you will have gray hair. If you have a bit of pheomelanin and brown eumelanin, you'll have strawberry blond hair. Combinations of these three pigments are what create the many shades of color we see throughout the different people in the world.

There is no actual blue or green pigment anywhere in the human

---

i. *Polymorphous light eruption.*

body, and you will be hard pressed to find blue anywhere in nature. Due to the way light is reflected inside the eye, they might appear various shades of blue and green. In the same way the ocean appears different shades of blue or green depending on the scene playing out above it, blue eyes—even the feathers of a bright blue bird—have no blue in them at all. They are merely reflecting a select portion of the light that is hitting them, giving us the perception that they are blue. If you were to grind the feathers of the brightest blue bird into smaller particles, the feathers would no longer be blue—not because they lost their blue pigment, but because they lost their structural ability to reflect back select portions of the color spectrum.

These two types of melanin—eumelanin and pheomelanin—are produced from exposure to UV radiation from the sun. Melanin is very effective at diffusing and blocking these UV rays. If you receive a lot of sunlight, your body will produce melanin in your newest skin cells and you will appear to be darker. Because your body is constantly shedding old skin cells, your tan will fade without maintaining sun exposure.

If you look at a map of the world that overlays the predominant skin color of native populations, a pattern will be visible: Lighter skinned people live further away from the equator. Similarly, the closer you get to the equator, the darker their skin becomes. The reason for this is not a hotly debated topic—most will say the body is creating additional protection to ensure the skin is not severely damaged. It makes sense, at first.

Towards the equator is more direct sunlight, and the native populations of these latitudes create melanin more aggressively to prevent skin damage. Higher latitude people also create melanin to protect their skin, but with the UV radiation less pronounced in their locales, they do not need to create as much and as a result, their skin is lighter.

Some will point to studies showing there is less skin cancer amongst indigenous, darker-skinned equatorial inhabitants. While this may seem reasonable, one must ask: If the equatorial populations are creating enough melanin to keep their skin from damage, then why aren't the others? Sure there are differences based on location, but relatively speaking, shouldn't the melanin efforts of a New Englander be just as sufficient for protection as the people of Uganda or Kenya?

Obviously, there are genetic components to skin color that no amount of sun exposure or avoidance will modify, but when you notice someone's ability to tan change drastically within their lifetime—within the course of perhaps a few months—you cannot help but feel that some core function of their body has changed.

For those who have lost their ability to tan, I suspect their body mistakenly believes that it's deficient in vitamin D and is desperately trying to *stop* producing melanin. Their body is making every adjustment it can to allow more sunlight through the skin and into the *7-Dehydrocholesterol* inside—a process it hopes which will lead to the creation of more vitamin D. Besides reducing their ability to tan, a decrease in melanin will create a dramatic shift in skin tone, and can even cause their eyes to change hue—as illustrated in the story above.

Elevated levels of vitamin D are normally handled with ease. You will probably never see someone's skin tone become darker in an attempt to lower their vitamin D production. But the opposite frequently happens. In an immune system that is being taken over with intracellular infections, the body mistakenly believes it needs more vitamin D and modulates everything it can to fix the problem—even turning a golden bronzed girl into a lily-white flower.

If you are able to get the chronic infections in your body under control, I would expect your body's vitamin D processes to normalize, which will cause melanin production to return to its normal level.

Although it may seem like a trivial loss compared to the many other things you may suffer, the healthy skin tone you remember from the summers of your childhood may not be so far away.

FEMALES & AUTOIMMUNITY

Through study of man-made disease, an obvious question will arise: Why do females have 78% of autoimmune diseases?[202] Males tend to develop more neurological issues early on as children, but females get many more autoimmune disorders—often starting in their teens and 20s. With so many people suffering, it is an inquiry that doesn't get the allocation of research funds that prevention, healing and cures might. Regardless, I feel behind every strange pattern is a clue that can help unravel the unknown—and this mystery may offer a big one.

If immune activation events are the triggers for man-made disease, then females are already likely to win the race. Between monthly cycles and pregnancy, a female's body chemistry offers far more opportunities for immunological disruption. The endometrium that females develop every month provides additional receptors for vitamin D to work its sometimes deleterious effects.[203] In a natural state, this should provide them with additional immunological protection, but as we've seen with vitamin D and a body in a chronic state of inflammation, this increase in vitamin D receptors can have the opposite effect—giving intracellular bacteria an additional surface through which they can disrupt the immune system.[204] In a body filled with metal or possibly antibiotics, this presents a monthly opportunity for intracellular bacteria to start a new infection or regain any ground they had lost in the previous few weeks.

Another reason females may develop more autoimmune disease than men has to do with the granulomas. The rise and fall in estrogen, progesterone, and more specifically the relaxin hormone may be causing the breakdown of the tissue that make up the granulomas. Studies have shown how relaxin can reduce the fibrous growths of fibrosis,[205] so it isn't hard to imagine its effects on granulomas. Similar to the physical exertion so often linked with the onset of these diseases, granulomas—which had safely sequestered the metals away—may become less rigid due to the influence of these hormones and eventually collapse, triggering a release of aluminum into the bloodstream or lymphatic system.

Most males do not experience autoimmune disease in their teens like this. Although very young boys experience more neurological effects from metal—an effect explained in the autism chapters—males do not have as much of an autoimmune problem. Not only are their granuloma formations more likely to be more robust, they do not have a monthly hormone coursing through their body which is designed to break down tissue.

There is a reason why so many perfectly healthy girls begin to experience "autoimmune" issues in their mid-teens, and I don't think it's only because they suddenly became very physically active. While exertion may significantly affect the integrity of granuloma formation and promote the redistribution of aluminum, I believe the hormonal influence of relaxin from their monthly cycle is the culprit. After a few years of pressure, relaxin can break down the granulomas that had been safely storing the metal, releasing it into the blood and lymphatic system.

By itself, this event is not enough to create autoimmune illness. However, once aluminum has collected in these areas, the next time a girl develops an infection like strep or Mono, the cycle of chronic infection might begin. The wrong antibiotics may be administered and it will become a very big problem. If you have a young daughter who was fully vaccinated and appears in perfect health, you may want to consider starting aluminum chelation now to lessen the chance of some of these autoimmune diseases from happening.

PARKINSON'S

In many of the diseases we have discussed, I have looked for their analog amongst the medical literature of the 1800s, when medicinal metals began to be administered so heavily. Parkinson's disease, first described more than 100 years before Dr. Alzheimer was treating Auguste Deter, is different—its peculiar symptoms first appeared in 1817 and the original name still exists.

Parkinson's has a few unique characteristics that make it stand out from some of the other neurodegenerative diseases: slowed movement, muscle weakness, and tremors, even at rest. Other symptoms such as cognitive decline, memory problems and hallucinations overlap, but there is enough of a difference that a separate diagnosis can be made, particularly in later stages of the disease.

The main difference in Parkinson's disease and Alzheimer's is the location inside the brain which it affects. The damage seen in Parkinson's is confined to a very specific area—the *substantia nigra,* which means "dark substance." In a previous chapter on tanning, I said there were three types of melanin but only mentioned two—

eumelanin, which give us black and brown pigments, and pheomelanin, which gives us red. The third type of melanin is a special type of pigment called *neuromelanin*. It doesn't color the skin or tissues we can easily see—it colors the brain.

Although many structures in the brain run together and can't be easily distinguished without sophisticated staining methods, the substantia nigra stands out because it is full of the neuromelanin pigment, giving it its dark color. The substantia nigra is responsible for the production of dopamine. If there is a loss of dopamine in the brain, it begins to function poorly, losing its ability for motor planning, speech, and sleep, among other problems—many of the hallmark symptoms of Parkinson's.

The fact that Parkinson's brains are showing signs of aluminum in the substantia nigra should surprise no one.[206] Additionally, researchers have been able to create Parkinson's-like behaviors in rats with chronic dietary exposure to aluminum.[207] Like Alzheimer's disease, anti-inflammatory medicines seem to have a protective effect on the development of Parkinson's. Even forty years ago scientists had already realized that increased dietary aluminum could lead to lower levels of dopamine[208] but didn't understand why.

The purpose of neuromelanin is still unclear, but it does appear to do one thing very well—chelate metal. Using a sophisticated laser, researchers detected both iron and aluminum in the neuromelanin in Parkinson's patients while finding no evidence of metal in the neuromelanin of those without the disease.[209] While its interaction with iron—a natural substance within the body—may serve a useful purpose, containing aluminum comes at a cost. Parkinson's patients have much less neuromelanin as other patients[210] and the mechanism by which these cells can be destroyed by aluminum has been clearly illustrated.[211] With no other apparent purpose, it would appear that the neuromelanin serves no other function but to protect the substantia nigra from metal toxicity.

The substantia nigra—and the neuromelanin within—both have special traits that make for a particularly unfortunate combination. It would appear that neuromelanin can chelate iron without problems, but with aluminum, the chelation causes damage. For some reason, the immune-system cells within the substantia nigra—called *microglia*—react very strongly[212] to inflammation, a response so robust it frequently causes the death of the cells responsible for the production of dopamine.[213]

Like many of the other diseases and disorders we've looked at, the inflammation from this event is likely to attract more aluminum. The fact that the area of the brain associated with Parkinson's has a natural chelator might seem to be good news. An increase in the amount of the chelator—neuromelanin—might also seem good. Unfortunately, neuromelanin is good at binding aluminum, but the after effects may create an infinite cascade of inflammation that will not stop until there is no more metal left in the body.

You might be wondering something—if many of the symptoms of Parkinson's are caused by dopamine deficiency, why couldn't we just inject dopamine into the brain to offset the deficiency? As mentioned elsewhere, much of the brain is protected by something called the blood brain barrier—it's a second layer around the blood vessels. Very little can get through—by design. If you drilled a hole into the skull and injected dopamine directly inside, it would not be able to make use of the intricate distribution system within the brain—the blood vessels. Even if you injected it into the blood vessels serving the brain, it would just cycle through and eventually get used up somewhere else. This is what makes treating neurological disorders with medicine so difficult. The brain is very well protected from outside invaders, but as is the case with both aluminum and intracellular bacteria, they can easily get past this defense by hiding inside white blood cells.

Is Parkinson's simply Alzheimer's disease but with a slightly different initial site of inflammation? It would appear so. There is of course a genetic element to the equation—as there always is—that may predispose you to develop problems in this particular area of the brain, but whatever the case, genetics alone are not likely to be the cause.

While the chronic inflammation from Alzheimer's may require a microbe like *Chlamydophila pneumoniae,* the unique chelation and inflammatory features of the substantia nigra may not require it, a hypothesis supported by the scarcity of bacterial infections linked to Parkinson's.

Parkinson's disease is a horrible diagnosis for anyone and their caregivers to deal with. It appears that it may be simply due to metal toxicity in the brain. As our abilities to safely remove aluminum from the body increase—along with our more careful consumption of aluminum containing products—Parkinson's disease should fade into the history books.

PROGRESSIVE SUPRANUCLEAR PALSY

There is another neurodegenerative disease which closely resembles Parkinson's and Alzheimer's but differs in the area of the brain that it affects. I want to mention its description—see if you can guess the location of neurological damage:

> "...an uncommon brain disorder that affects movement, control of walking (gait) and balance, speech, swallowing, vision, mood and behavior, and thinking... One of the classic signs of the disease is an inability to aim and move the eyes properly, which individuals may experience as blurring of vision."[214]

If this cluster of symptoms sounds familiar to you, then you are probably familiar with many of the problems common amongst cranial nerve palsies. Gait and balance issues can be caused by 9th cranial nerve problems. Speech, by the 12th, 5th and 7th. Swallowing by the 9th and 10th. Vision by the 2nd, 3rd and 6th. Mood and behavior issues by the 10th. *Progressive supranuclear palsy* (PSP) is a terrible disease for which there is no known cause or cure. It is very rare, but like many of the other unexplained neurological diseases, treatment is often palliative at best.

The disease is called progressive for obviously unfortunate reasons. Supranuclear indicates the damage occurs above the cranial nerve nuclei, frequently the 3rd oculomotor cranial nerve nuclei. Damage in this location causes one of the most common symptoms of the disease —trouble looking down.

"The first and second wrecks were fender benders, but the third one was really bad," someone whose mother had passed away from this disease told me.

His mother was a beautiful, vibrant woman who, having emigrated to the United States from eastern Europe, took nothing for granted. She was having difficulty controlling her eyes, and had gotten into her third car wreck within a few short years.

"She had always been so outgoing—any social function that came her way—she would go. I noticed her not going out as much and just chalked it up to getting a little older."

Though his mother was only 55 at the time, other troubling signs began to appear. Things that felt wrong for someone so young.

"Whenever we visited, she would always have huge spreads of food —she loved cooking. The spreads got smaller and smaller. Again—little warning signs that seem obvious looking back. But then her fridge started getting more and more empty, and I remember looking at some of the jars inside and noticed they were expired. It's funny how a little thing like that stands out—there were other things that were obviously wrong—but the expired food—that one little thing was when I started researching what might be wrong with her."

His mother would decline slowly over the next eight years until she finally passed away, but the specific symptoms of her illness were unmistakable.

"She had problems with her eyes, and I remember her face—her mouth not being even, like Bell's Palsy or something. She had trouble drinking out of that side of her mouth, but then she had trouble even swallowing towards the end—that was a horrible thing to see."

This rare disease is often initially diagnosed as Parkinson's disease. Progressive supranuclear palsy lacks the tremors common in Parkinson's but has many similarities: stiffness, clumsiness, and difficulties with movement. But it is the other symptoms that make awareness of this disease so important.

When children experience any of the issues common to PSP, such as difficulty swallowing, vision problems, motion disorders or behavioral issues, most doctors will throw their hands up in the air.

"We don't know what causes this," they'll sometimes say with a shrug of the shoulders. But if you were to suggest to them that your child's issues are simply caused by lesions around the cranial nerve nuclei within their brain stem—they would likely dismiss it as wild speculation.

Because progressive supranuclear palsy is often fatal, the opportunities for neurological scrutiny are plentiful. The resulting research has made it clear—the symptoms of PSP are caused by the deterioration of brain cells in a particular area—the brain stem, specifically the cranial nerve nuclei. Why this same area is not suspected as a possible source for the cause of similar symptoms in children is odd.

Progressive supranucelar palsy is thankfully a rare disease. But its peculiar set of symptoms, coupled with anatomical studies that have made clear where the problem begins, should be an enormous arrow in the sky, pointing towards the cranial nerve nuclei in the brain stem. This is where many of the unexplainable disorders we see in children today are originating from.

THYROID & HASHIMOTO'S

Thyroid conditions are thought to be the most common autoimmune disorders. Fatigue and unexplained weight gain. Cold fingers and toes. Hair falling out. The thyroid hormone affects nearly everything in your body, and without enough of it, the effects can be debilitating. Despite its frequent occurrence, many people suffer silently for years before realizing their thyroid is the cause of their problems.

The most common issue with your thyroid happens when it doesn't produce enough of the thyroid hormone. Occasionally, it will produce too much, but a deficit is more common. When the thyroid is producing too little and there is no obvious cause, it will often be labeled Hashimoto's syndrome—an autoimmune-caused hypothyroidism.

Chronic inflammation can begin to destroy your thyroid gland and prevent it from producing enough hormone for your body. Like all autoimmune disorders, the mechanism by which this happens is not completely understood, but has been associated with the aluminum adjuvants in vaccines.[215]

To complicate matters, thyroid antibodies—the thing they test Hashimoto's for—are present in up to 25% of people with type 1 diabetes and over half of them go on to develop some form of autoimmune thyroid disease.[216] Thyroid antibodies are so plentiful that far more people have thyroid antibodies than have thyroid disease. It would appear that thyroid antibodies are not the distinct marker we would like—something else may be suppressing the function of this gland.

By now, a pattern of vitamin D deficiency has emerged in many of these autoimmune disorders, and hypothyroidism is no different.[217] While most interpret vitamin D deficiency as contributing to autoimmunity, I believe it is the direct result of a dysfunctioning immune system.[i]

A new school of thought is emerging in the study of autoimmune disorders that may point even more strongly to this. Many of the immune cells in your body have vitamin D receptors on them, called VDR. There are over sixty different types of these receptors, and their job is to dock with vitamin D and send out instructions to your immune system. The intracellular bacteria can block these receptors and create havoc in your immune response. It is very poorly understood as to why, but for some reason, certain types of these receptors appear to be associated with Hashimoto's thyroiditis—an autoimmune response to your thyroid.[218]

I am going to hypothesize here quite a bit—much further than I am comfortable doing elsewhere. If certain types of VDR are actively being blocked by intracellular bacteria, it could disrupt the coordinated response your body is designed to create. In this scenario, intracellular bacteria are causing the VDR blockage, but a viral infection could

---

i. Read the chapter "The Problem with Vitamin D" for a more thorough explanation.

trigger the improper response—a sequence of events that may explain how intracellular bacteria can negatively affect your body's immune response to viral infections.

This is important because autoimmune thyroid diseases are more frequently associated with viruses than bacteria.[219] While chronic inflammation from a bacterial infection could certainly cause hypothyroidism, I believe something different may be going on—a disruptive immune response to a viral infection due to VDR blockage by the intracellular bacteria. The end result is the same—chronic inflammation of a vital organ or gland in the body, but with a slightly different twist—this time it's the bacteria and virus working together to cause problems.

Whatever the cause, I don't believe autoimmune diseases are an unrelenting curse laid upon you by a poor genetic lottery ticket. The mechanisms that cause autoimmune conditions should be able to be reversed. Fortunately, the same techniques discussed in the healing and recovery chapter of this book should work to repair your immune system and break the cycle of inflammation.

MULTIPLE SCLEROSIS

Multiple sclerosis (MS) is considered an autoimmune disease. Most people develop subtle symptoms like an occasional tingle in their foot that comes and goes or fogginess in one of their eyes. The illness can progress to debilitating stages of pain and paralysis. The symptoms are caused by damage to the *myelin*—an electrical layer of insulation that surrounds connections between parts of your brain called *axons*. Myelin is an amazing substance in that it helps propagate electrical signals through the axons in your brain—even protecting other messages from crossing over and interfering.

If you develop enough damage to the myelin, your nerves will not fire correctly and the problem will be visible as lesions on your brain in an MRI. Because your brain is full of axons, these issues can affect the function of nearly any part of your body. While the nerve pains and vision problems associated with multiple sclerosis can be horrible, one of the most common debilitating traits of the disorder is fatigue—extreme, full body tiredness not unlike that seen in chronic fatigue syndrome. Lesions in the hypothalamus might easily cause the disruptions these people experience[220] but could also be triggered elsewhere.

At this point, any time you see unexplained neurological damage anywhere in someone's central nervous system, you should look for signs of metal toxicity. If a disorder is described as "autoimmune," you should double your efforts. The lesions in multiple sclerosis appear to be the direct result of aluminum toxicity. In fact, not only does aluminum damage myelin, it would seem to have a preference for it.[221]

We know that compared to people with no signs of neurodegenerative damage, MS patients show elevated levels of aluminum (and other metals) in their urine after taking chelation drugs designed to eliminate them from their body.[222] And perhaps even more telling, an MS patient who hadn't responded to traditional medication responded well to chelation. As they measured increased amounts of aluminum, lead and mercury in his urine, his MS symptoms improved.[223]

Like Alzheimer's disease, MS is associated with chronic inflammation of microglia—the immune cells of the brain.[224] With Alzheimer's, there are just a few bacterial infections that appear to be associated. Although scientists are fairly certain there is a viral or bacterial component to multiple sclerosis, the search for a single microbe has not yielded any answers. A study looked for Epstein-Barr virus—the subject of frequent MS associations—in the lesions of 21 multiple sclerosis patients, but found none.[225] Another bacteria commonly associated with MS—*Chlamydia pneumoniae* – was found in only 2.9% of MS patients and in none of the controls.[226]

The antiquated quest for a single pathogen causing a single illness will continue to vex researchers because with multiple sclerosis, like many other man-made diseases, there is probably not a single pathogen involved. Any microbe—viral or bacterial—capable of inflammation can summon aluminum-containing white blood cells to that area of the body.

Understanding which bacteria or viruses can be safely used with certain antibiotics without creating cell-wall deficient forms is important to advance the state of medicine. Trying to pin down which bacteria or virus causes which man-made disease may prove to be an exercise in futility, but for the curious scientist, it may help understand how metals and microbes interact to create various forms of inflammation. We will never create bodies without microbes—and indeed, we shouldn't try. But a body without metal—that is a noble pursuit we should all work towards.

We know that MS is the result of environmental variables in your life—genetically speaking, only 1 in 3 identical twins will develop MS if the other twin already has it.[227] This would indicate that the amount of metal you have in your body and the types of microbial infections you've experienced are far more indicative of whether you are likely to develop the lesions of multiple sclerosis.

There are studies that indicate head trauma may increase your chances of getting multiple sclerosis, an unsurprising correlation with any neurodegenerative disease once you understand the connection between inflammation and metal. Similarly, in light of what we know about the way chronic infections can manipulate your body's use of vitamin D, it's unsurprising that in a body full of metal scientists might associate multiple sclerosis with problems metabolizing vitamin D[228]— hypotheses which have until now been missing a few important pieces.

Although the suffering it causes is horrible, multiple sclerosis is a simple disease of metals and microbes. Infections, stress, and even head trauma will create the inflammation that draw metals into the brain where the myelin sheaths that cover the axons represent an irresistible target to any aluminum that happens to come in contact with them. In a world without ingested or injected metal, multiple sclerosis would not exist.

ECZEMA

Unlike many of the other illnesses mentioned in this book, eczema-like conditions appear to have existed throughout history. Scabies—an infection with a name that sounds as horrible as the illness—is caused by tiny mites that burrow into your skin and lay their eggs. Another skin illness—hand, foot and mouth disease—can be caused by a variety of pathogens. Other infections are known to cause problems such as the *Eczema Coxsackium* seen in coxsackievirus A6 outbreaks—a reaction so intense it is referred to as a case of "serious" hand, foot and mouth disease. *Eczema vaccinatum*, a life threatening skin condition, was accepted as a risk of the frequently contaminated smallpox vaccine.

As you read through the history of eczema, one thing stands out—it is associated with a viral or bacterial infection. It typically comes and goes with the appearance and disappearance of illness. Infants would occasionally develop problems, but like their parents, it would go away once the infection had cleared.

There is a seemingly infinite variety of eczema lesions: macules, patches, vesicles and plaques. Like the myriad cloud formations meteorologists study, the variety of outbreaks of eczema could always be described more precisely if given enough time. Whatever the shape or size of your eczema, I believe they are the result of a long-running infection within your body. They are the same skin lesions of old, but with a modern twist—your body cannot get rid of the infection causing them. They will come and go with the rise and fall of your immune system—sometimes with an obvious trigger like stress or illness, other times seemingly out of nowhere.

Just like some infections have a propensity for the throat or intestines, others may thrive in the areas just under the skin. The location of your breakouts may seem like a complete mystery, but areas of the skin where there is greater friction and sub-clinical inflammation —even though you would never think of them as such—may bear the brunt of the problem.

There are some that have seen dietary changes affect their breakouts and assume this meant their eczema was the manifestation of a food allergy. Interestingly, an exhaustive 400-page book from 1901 titled "Eczema With an Analysis of Eight Thousand Cases of the Disease"[229] mentions nothing about food allergies. Why? Because food allergies would not exist for at least another forty years.

This doesn't prove that eczema isn't caused by food allergies, but alterations in your diet may actually just promote healthy gut bacteria —an action which will tip the immune system into a state less favorable to breakouts.[230] Studies have confirmed that probiotics can have positive effects on eczema.[231] The role of the good bacteria in your gut is not completely understood, but one thing they appear to do is proliferate in such numbers that they essentially form a protective coating over the intestine that prevents other potentially harmful bacteria from thriving.

There are certainly rashes and hives associated with food allergies, but I believe those are different lesions than the persistent, weeks and months long outbreaks of eczema. You might occasionally see a group of small white circles on your skin that feel rough and painless. These are probably not eczema at all but harmless fungal infections that may benefit from a metallic environment in the same way bacteria do.

In a body without metal, infections could be cleared completely and you might never see a particular type of outbreak again. In the new age of chronic infection, you may see a frequent breakout completely disappear, only to resurface years later after the flu or a difficult fight with your significant other.

To those who haven't suffered the pain or stigma of a face covered in a breakout, eczema may seem like a minor inconvenience that can be treated with some cream from the grocery store. Those who've experienced this condition, and live in fear each day it will return at the worst possible moment—like a wedding day or job interview—know how much this "simple" illness can change your life. While I cannot say for sure if this is what is causing eczema, I believe it is likely the culprit —long-running infections which occasionally surface in this painful way. Getting rid of the metal which enables these long-running infections, then clearing out the leftover bacteria and viruses should allow you to live the rest of your life without more outbreaks.

ANEMIA

Like heart disease, issues with the blood may seem like a strange place to look for the effects of metals and microbes. It is common sense that tissues, organs, even the brain can suffer the effects of inflammation, but the blood itself seems like a neutral player in this battle—transporting things around your body, but not itself under assault. I know several people who suffer the debilitating effects of anemia and even though many of them also experience other symptoms of chronic inflammation, I was skeptical there was any link. Regardless, I began looking through the scientific literature and was amazed at what I found.

Anemia refers to a condition in which someone has either fewer red blood cells than normal or the red blood cells themselves have a decreased ability to deliver oxygen. The symptoms of anemia can range from shortness of breath, heart palpitations to *pica*—the eating of things with no nutritional value such as ice. Low iron levels are not just the domain of adults—they are also a common marker in children with autism,[232] Asperger syndrome,[233] and even ADHD.[234]

Aluminum itself is also associated with anemia, particularly the anemia that patients who are undergoing dialysis often experience from the metal contained in their dialysis fluid.[235] The process is poorly understood, but may be connected to another blood disorder called *neutropenia*. This disorder is characterized by abnormally low values of white blood cells called neutrophils and can lead not only to frequent infections, but more severe infections as their immune system is unequipped to fight them properly. Antibiotics and intracellular bacteria may play a role in this condition and have been studied.[236]

The chronic inflammation as described in this book can also cause anemia through a well-understood process—it creates elevated *Interleukin-6*, a protein which affects the way iron is absorbed through the body. Without enough iron in the blood cells, they will lose their ability to carry oxygen and their red coloring. With chronic inflammation, you will feel the changes in your body caused by this iron issue and in fact, you will even be able to see it as your skin color turns less red and more yellow.

Your hematologist may acknowledge the symptoms you have related but look with confusion at the results from your blood panels. Why? Your iron levels may be slightly off, but not enough to create the dramatic effects you are experiencing. With the clock on the wall ticking and without an obvious answer, they will suggest you need more iron. You could receive bag after bag of iron transfusions, sitting for hours in the recliner alongside the chemo patients, but your symptoms will not improve.

This may be because iron deficiency is not the actual problem. Your body may be incapable of using the iron it already has due to the elevated Interleukin-6 levels produced by chronic inflammation raging in your body. The iron transfusions may help a bit, but they will miss the mark. Your doctor may not be aware of this phenomenon and is unlikely to ask for a simple SED rate or C-Reactive Protein test that might indicate the source of the problem.

For someone who is already sick from the effects of multiple infections in their body, this relatively unknown side-effect of chronic inflammation does little to improve the situation. If you are able to get the intracellular infections in your body under control, you should see many anemia related symptoms disappear.

HEART DISEASE

Heart attacks and other forms of heart disease seem unlikely to be affected by aluminum or antibiotics. It's tempting to believe that heart disease has been around since the beginning of time and will always be a presence among the unlucky few. I expect heart attacks have existed for a very long time, but the frequency and relative health or youth of many of those stricken down should give anyone pause before they dismiss someone's death as inevitable.

Mechanically speaking, heart attacks most often happen because of the loss of blood flow into the heart. Other common problems involve damage to the structural integrity of the organ itself, but the most common issue is not enough blood going into the heart. How could the presence of metal in the body or antibiotic use contribute to heart disease?

Remember that aluminum is a toxin whose very presence can destroy cells. This is a particular problem in neuronal tissue, where aluminum is especially destructive. Alzheimer's and other neurodegenerative diseases appear to happen when aluminum and the chronic inflammation associated with bacterial infections meet. A similar effect may be responsible for some heart disease.

For instance, a common bacteria called C. pneumoniae has often been found in the blood of elderly patients who have suffered from a stroke.[237] What's more concerning is the discovery of this bacteria directly in the atherosclerotic plaques of coronary artery disease patients.[238] As plaque builds up in your arteries, blood flow returning to your heart is impaired. Why would particular bacteria be found so often within these plaques?

Another study looked at C. pneumonia, H. pylori and C-reactive protein, a common marker of inflammation and found similarly disturbing results.[239] Both bacteria indicated a 2.5 times higher risk for *acute myocardial infarction*[i] than those without the bacteria. Those with raised levels of C-reactive protein, a less specific measurement of inflammation, had a 3.85 times higher risk. These are not isolated studies—there are numerous papers correlating bacterial infections with these problems.

Heart disease is often thought of as the result of predetermined genetic markers alongside a few environmental factors. Smoking and obesity are often listed as two risk factors for heart disease, but these studies begin to make you wonder—are they just two more sources of inflammation adding to the mix?

Could the chronic inflammation caused by aluminum and antibiotic use be unwittingly causing damage to the lining of the blood vessels, a condition that accelerates the buildup of plaque in coronary heart disease? It might seem like an implausible idea, but when studies are finding C. pneumonia in the plaques that cause heart attacks, the possible association becomes difficult to ignore.

Myocarditis is another debilitating heart disease marked by inflammation and damage to the muscle. Unlike heart disease,

---

i. Heart attack.

myocarditis seems to occur in perfectly healthy, athletic, non-smoking people. In males, the average age of onset is between 16-20 years old.[240] And like heart attacks and coronary artery disease, myocarditis is frequently associated with bacterial, sometimes viral infections.

Could chronic inflammation from unseen bacterial infections be the source of aggravation that cause myocarditis to develop? The body's immune system can normally take care of an infection within a few days. What might cause a long-running chronic infection that could lead to heart failure? I can't think of anything other than intracellular bacteria and the vicious circle of inflammation they cause. By itself, your body's immune system would be able to kill them off. With the presence of aluminum and possibly antibiotics, they can survive and thrive for years despite your body's best efforts.

As we move forward in our understanding of heart attacks, coronary artery disease and myocarditis, it would make sense that we consider the role of metal and antibiotics in their development. There's a reason healthy 20-year-olds have heart attacks, and it's not just a genetic fluke.

HEALING & RECOVERY

Pull the weeds and the garden will grow.

FIRST STEPS

Most modern medicine focuses on alleviating symptoms, rather than treating the underlying cause. For many of the man-made diseases, they don't know the cause so it's understandable they would attempt to treat the symptoms—it's better than nothing.

The most important step in healing from man-made disease is realizing something you may have already begun to do: your or your children's health is your responsibility. Completely. Totally. You have more time to invest in understanding these illnesses. You have more at stake than any doctor or behavioral therapist. Although they are important partners and may have more knowledge than you do, your desire to get better will eclipse nearly anything someone else can offer you.

Unless you are extremely fortunate and can find a physician who is already onboard with this concept of man-made disease, you will need to understand these concepts enough to get your doctor excited about it. The good news is the methods suggested in this book are thoroughly supported by scientific research.

Healing from man-made disease can be challenging—it is not just a simple diet change or regimen of pills. You will need to become familiar with some new concepts and become comfortable working alongside your physician. You will need to be in-tune with your body and learn to make adjustments along the way.

Thankfully, the underlying cause of man-made disease may be very simple. I believe it comes down to two things:

1) Acute metal toxicity.
2) Chronic inflammation.

It's my belief that modern healing and recovery methods should focus on determining if the disorder is purely due to metal toxicity or if there is also a chronic infection involved. Determining between these two will provide you with the information you need to begin healing.

There are conditions mentioned in this book that may have caused permanent damage that is irreversible, and I don't want to give someone false hope where there may be little. Neurological disorders can be difficult to reverse if the damage has been occurring for a long time. However, one of the greatest miracles of the human body is in its ability to heal. It is designed to mend itself, especially in its natural state. If you have metal toxicity and/or chronic inflammation—these are two unnatural conditions that will prevent your body from healing. In fact, nearly all of the diseases mentioned in this book may actually be just symptoms of your body trying to heal itself. Nearly all modern disease can potentially be prevented, if not healed, by two things:

1) Get rid of the metal in your body.
2) Get rid of the chronic inflammation in your body.

If you can do these two things, the body may begin to recover from many of the disorders listed in this book. I am not suggesting that complete recovery is possible from every disease, no matter the severity. But the sooner you can get started addressing these two problems, the more likely complete recovery is possible.

You will probably need to find a licensed physician who can work together with you. This may take some searching—integrative doctors in your area are a good place to start. There is also a term called "functional medicine" that may help you find an open-minded health care provider who is willing to think inside a different box than they're used to.

While there are many remedies that may work at your local health food store—from natural anti-microbials to high dose vitamins—you are probably reading this chapter right now because you or someone you love has a big problem—a man-made problem that has put the body and immune system in a very unnatural state. I wish that I could go into my backyard and grow the components needed to heal from these issues. Maybe, one day, we will discover a way to do this.

For now, I believe there are certain scenarios where man-made problems may require man-made fixes. If you or your loved one is very sick, you may not have enough time to use the gentle five-year techniques that nature has provided us—you may need something that works faster, even if there is a small amount of risk.

For that reason, you will need to partner with a physician who understands chelation, antibiotics and is willing to learn a few new things about the way the immune system and chronic infections work. Don't worry, there is a specific plan I am going to recommend for you and your doctor to work through—it is staffed by incredible volunteers and is thoroughly supported by scientific research.

METAL TOXICITY

The first step in beginning to prevent or heal from most of these modern diseases is to get rid of the metal in your body. This is not an easy task. Metal was never supposed to be ingested or injected and consequently, our body is not very good at getting it out. It gets into organs like the liver or brain. Even when it's not actively harming us, our body can store it inside granulomas under the skin and deep within muscle tissue.

Permanently getting rid of chronic infection in your body is going to be very difficult until the metal comes out. All of your progress can be instantly set back because of the metal. So take this step seriously— the metal has to come out or your immune system will not have a fair battle against the microbes it will encounter.

Avoiding metal

Before starting the long process of getting rid of metal in your body, you need to learn the common environmental sources of metal and make sure to avoid them. Environmental metal can come from things like aluminum pans, cookware, certain antiperspirants, antacids, cosmetic mineral oils, and even some water supplies. Seafood can contain a lot of metal—if this is a food you enjoy, you should do some research on what is safe to eat and may want to consider limiting your intake.

Medicinal metals are probably the largest source of metal in a child born today. Many of the vaccines they receive contain large amounts of aluminum. The DTaP shot, which they are likely to receive at least five times, contains 350 micrograms of aluminum. The Hepatitis B shot they are likely to receive at birth contains 250 micrograms of aluminum.

If the thought of not giving your child any vaccines that contain aluminum scares you as much as giving them aluminum—you are not alone. Many parents are terrified at skipping shots for their children. A growing number of parents are opting for "vaccine alternatives" because of their concern about the ingredients. These parents would never consider themselves "anti-vaxxers", but are simply trying to make long-term investment in the health of their children. Scientific research is helping them find safer, more natural ways to prevent their children from getting and/or spreading disease.

Removing mercury

There are many different ways to remove metal from your body. It can be dangerous and is a process that should not be lightly considered. Thankfully, there is a very thoroughly-researched metal chelation method that I have personally seen create huge steps towards recovery. And for those of you with older children, I believe it is never too late to start getting metal out of their body. I have heard that even teenagers may show neurological improvements after undergoing dedicated metal chelation therapies.

For mercury toxicity, a technique which comes up often is called the Andy Cutler protocol. It is a very specific protocol that requires frequent administration of the medicine every few hours for a couple of days at a time—even through the night. This can be especially challenging if you're administering it to fussy children who already have sleep disorders, but again, many of the people who have stuck with it have seen progress. This protocol is not just for children, and can be used by any adult with chronic inflammation issues. Even if you are completely unvaccinated, you are unlikely to have a body free of metal.

Mercury may be less of a problem due to its increasing rarity within vaccines, but because of maternal transfer and other environmental sources, it is difficult to say whether you or your child may have mercury toxicity. Even the testing itself can be contentious, as some say that hair tests with low mercury levels may simply indicate an inability to naturally chelate mercury out of the body.

If you have metal amalgams in your mouth you should begin saving some money to have them safely removed. This is an extremely toxic process that a classically-trained dentist is unlikely to do correctly. Make sure you find a dentist who uses special filtration systems and a dental dam in your mouth during the procedure. If they are only charging you a hundred dollars per amalgam, it's too cheap—look for someone else. Do not even think about trying to save money by having an uninformed dentist perform this procedure—I have spoken to a few women who developed intense "autoimmune" diseases after having their amalgams improperly removed. They would have been better off leaving them in. The release of vapor from this operation is the most toxic form of mercury there is and needs to be done with extreme caution.

Removing aluminum

If you or your children are suffering the signs of acute neurological damage or chronic infection, I would think it's safe to say there is a metal toxicity problem. Increasingly, this is likely to be more from aluminum than mercury. Injected aluminum is in a form that may not be removed as well by mercury chelation techniques. There are differing opinions on this, as aluminum is thought by some to bind with mercury and will come out with traditional chelation.

There are a few chelation techniques for aluminum that you should familiarize yourself with. An easy one is *silica water*. In the United States, you can get it from a health food store or by buying Fiji® bottled water. The high silica levels in this water have an affinity for aluminum and will help your body excrete it. This is scientifically verified, by multiple studies. For instance, Alzheimer patients have shown improvements simply by drinking silica water. Many of us have gotten so used to believing if it doesn't come in a pill bottle then it can't actually work, but silica water will without a doubt work to remove metal from your body. It is a very slow process, and I would not expect results for weeks, if not months.

Glycine is an amino acid that can be found in certain foods or ingested in pill form. It serves many important functions within the body but has also been found to bind with aluminum and help your body excrete it. I would consider developing a daily regimen of silica water and glycine for anyone in your family who has been injected with aluminum.

Taurine, Lecithin and *Vitamin E* appear to have protective effects on the body from aluminum toxicity. Their ability to work as chelators is limited, but if you are in a situation where you must receive an aluminum-containing vaccine, such as a government job or the military, you may want to look into supplementing your diet with these three things.

The main problem in getting rid of aluminum is the persistent granulomas that may have formed throughout the body. It is impossible to say, but granulomas may protect the aluminum from the most aggressive forms of chelation. This is not encouraging, but is a reality we all need to face as we attempt to prevent long-term neurological damage seen with Alzheimer's and Parkinson's. It is unlikely that purposefully disturbing the granulomas and chelating the aluminum while it is circulating in the blood and lymphatic system will be a popular technique. Methods for safely removing the aluminum captured in granulomas will need to be developed and perfected.

HEALING CHRONIC INFECTION

With the metals coming out of your body, you can begin to fine tune the inflammation in your immune system and give your body a chance to heal from the chronic infections caused by intracellular bacteria. Remember that the metals may be a big reason these intracellular infections took root in your body to begin with, so while there is still metal present, it will be difficult to guarantee they won't come back.

If you feel like you may be suffering from chronic infection and want to get serious about helping your immune system get rid of it, there is a technique that many people have had success with. It is based on the Marshall protocol and employs particular antibiotics that do not cause bacteria to lose their cell wall. Instead, they target specifically intracellular forms. Combined with a very mild angiotensin inhibitor, this regimen will allow you to manipulate the way intracellular bacteria are able to interface with your immune system.

It is far too complex to attempt a simple explanation, but know that there are many people who have gone through this protocol and had remarkable success, even without the metal chelation component.

A team of volunteers runs the program at www.chronicillnessrecovery.org and will work with you and your physician to get you started on what they call "Inflammation Therapy." The people that run this site are medically trained, scientifically literate and have research papers to back up everything they suggest.

A quick word about antibiotics

Without getting too in-depth, I wanted to give you a quick overview of antibiotics because the wrong choice may make things worse. If you and your physician can work with the team at chronicillnessrecovery.org, they will help you decide which antibiotics are best for you. Regardless, you should familiarize yourself with the different types of antibiotics and their potential role in exacerbating chronic illness. **Consult with your physician on which antibiotics make the most sense for you.**

There are basically three types of antibiotics—*cell wall inhibitors, protein synthesis inhibitors* and *anti-malarial/anti-protozoals (cyst targeting antibiotics)*. The first kind, cell wall inhibitors, are generally not great antibiotics for dealing with intracellular infections. They promote the transformation of many bacteria into their other forms—the kind your immune system will have a more difficult time dealing with. In addition to attacking the bacteria itself, protein synthesis inhibitors can prevent bacteria from converting into intracellular forms and are sometimes better choices. The anti-malarial/anti-protozoal cyst targeting antibiotics can be effective, but will also produce the most side effects.

Cell wall inhibitors

Cephalosporins: Aztreonam (Azactam® for injection), Ceflacor

(Ceclor®), Cefadroxil (Duricef®), Cefamandole (Mandol®), Cefazolin (Ancef®, Kefzol®), Cefinir (Omnicef®), Cefepime (Maxipime®), Cefixime (Suprax®), Cefoperazone (Cefobid®), Cefotaxime (Claraforan®), Cefotetan (Cefotan®), Cefoxitin (Mefoxin®), Cefpodoxime (Vantin®), Cefprozil (Cefzil®), Ceftazidime (Ceptaz®, Fortaz®, Tazicef®, Tazidime®), Ceftibuten (Cedax®), Ceftozoxime (Cefizox®), **Ceftriaxone (Rocephin®)**, Cefuroxime (Ceftin®, Kefurox®, Zinacef®), Cephalexin (Keflex®, Keftab®), Cephapirin (Cephadyl®), Cephradine (Anspor®, Velocef®), Imipenem and Cilistatin (Primaxin I. V.®), Loracarbef (Lorabid®), and Meropenem (Merrem I.V.®)

Penicillins: Amoxicillin (Amoxil®, Trimox®), Amoxicillin and Clavulanate (Augmentin®), Ampicillin (Principen®, Totacillin®), Ampicillin and Sulbactam (Unisyn®), Bacampicillin (Spectrobid®), Carbenicillin (Geocillin®), Cloxacillin (Cloxapen®), Dicloxacillin (Dynapen®, Dycill®), Mezlocillin (Mezlin®), Nafcillin (Unipen®), Oxacillin (Bactocill®), Penicillin G (Bicillin C-R®, Bicillin L-A®, Pfizerpen®), Penicillin V (Beepen-VK®, Veetids®), Piperacillin (Pipracil®), Piperacillin and Tazobactam (Zosyn®), Ticarcillin (Ticar®), Ticarcillin and Clavulanate (Timentin®).

Protein Synthesis Inhibitors

Macrolides: Azithromycin (Zithromax®), clarithromycin (Biaxin®), dirithromycin (Dynabac®), roxythromycin (Rulid®).

Tetracyclines: Tetracycline, minocycline (Minocin®), Doxycycline.

Anti-malarials / Anti-protozoals / Cyst-form

Tinidazole (Fasigyn®), Metronidazole (Flagyl®), Secnidazole, Plaquenil®.

Antibiotics should be used sparingly and with the nature of the infection in mind. Anytime you use antibiotics you risk making the bacteria in your body resistant to it, so keep that in mind as you and your health team make decisions about which antibiotics to use.

SIGNS OF ACUTE METAL TOXICITY

I'm going to go over a few tests you can do that will allow you to watch for signs of metal toxicity in your children. Many times, parents may think they've noticed something change with their child after vaccines, but don't have a good reference point to determine what actually changed.

These tests should only take a few minutes but will offer you the peace of mind you are not imagining something changed (if something in fact, did). It may also give you the peace of mind knowing that perhaps your child hasn't changed at all, even though you may think it did.

If you are just reading this section without having read the rest of the book, the theory behind Crooked is that ingredients within vaccines, particularly the aluminum, can sometimes cause damage within the cranial nerves. Some of this damage may be difficult to diagnose in an infant who can't yet speak, but if you know what to look for, it can sometimes be visible on their face. Because you have two sets of each cranial nerve, one for the left and right sides of your body, problems with one may show up as asymmetry. If you do spot what might be cranial nerve damage after your children's shots, you may want to consider looking into healthy alternatives.

How to conduct these tests

I'm going to list some pointers that may make for the perfect testing scenario, but remember that anything is better than nothing. Many parents have been able to date the period something happened to their child based on pictures they randomly posted to Facebook, even though they had lost their phones and many of their photographs. So do you what you can—anything is better than nothing.

You should do these tests the day before your child gets their shots, then the day after, then a week after. Set reminders so you don't forget. You will need a camera, preferably one that can shoot slo-motion video, and preferably one with a flash on it. Your mobile phone will work perfectly.

Perform these tests when your child is alert and not eating. You need them attentive and without a mouth full of milk or food. It will also make comparison easier if you can shoot them in daylight hours near an uncovered window, though not in direct sunlight. The goal is to minimize shadows, as they can make a symmetrical face appear differently. As I mentioned earlier, anything is better than nothing, so if you're in the car in the parking lot of your pediatrician, you can make it work. Ideally, you will conduct these tests in the same location and lighting each time, something that will make comparison more accurate.

Also, it's often much easier to use video to catalog these tests rather than pictures. You can always go back later and take a screenshot of a particular frame from a paused video, rather than trying to take just the right picture. So if you have a phone that can shoot video, put the camera away and just shoot video.

One of the tests will be easier if you use the flash on your phone. The flash is not because things are too dark, but because the white dot created by the flash creates a registration marker on your child's eyes. The flash may be too bright for little ones. You can dim the flash by putting a piece or two of Scotch tape over the LED. Again, the brightness of the light is not particularly important—it's the reflection of the dot on their eye we need.

Dating these videos and pictures are important. Some phones allow you to quickly find the timestamp of when the video was recorded, but I've seen many pictures where for one reason or another, the parent can't accurately date the image. Sometimes parents will use an app to crop the photo or make a collage of images—these apps will strip the original timestamp from the image and make dating it difficult. For this reason, I'd suggest you save the original photos (if you take photos) and don't alter them in some other app. You need that original timestamp so that if something comes up, you can date them correctly.

One tip I recommend is that each time you start a test, clearly write the date on a piece of paper and take a picture of it before you start. Then, after your child gets their shots and you are taking the after pictures, write the date down again but this time list the shots they received. You can always find this information later, but it's much easier to do it now while it's fresh in your mind and you will have it right in sequence alongside images of their face.

What to do if these tests show something?

This is the part of any normal book where the author would advise the reader to consult with their physician about next steps to take. Unfortunately, I expect that not only will they not be able to explain why any of these symptoms have happened, they will also say it had nothing to do with their vaccines, suggest it will probably resolve itself, and finally send you home with more questions than answers, insisting that you need not be concerned.

The reason this book exists is specifically because: 1) parents are often very concerned when they notice these kinds of issues develop soon after vaccines were administered to their children and 2) I believe if one of these problems develop after vaccination, it may be a warning sign that your child is not able to handle the ingredients in the vaccines. I do recommend you mention what happened to your pediatrician, and show them the before/after image or video sequence to make your case.

Checking for 7th cranial nerve palsy

The 7th cranial nerves serve several purposes but are mainly used for controlling the muscles on your face. If your child develops lesions in one of their 7th cranial nerves it may be visible as three things:

1) A crooked smile.
2) The bottom of their mouth droops on one side.
3) Eyelids that don't close evenly.

You may not be able to make your baby spontaneously smile, but after you've written the date down on a piece of paper and taken a picture of it, take a video of your baby and do your best to get them to smile. Try to capture them smiling when they are looking straight at you. If you are able to catch them crying or frowning, make sure you capture video of this as well. Again, try to catch them looking straight at the camera.

In this test, you are looking for symmetry. Faces are rarely perfectly symmetrical when scrutinized at this level, and a little asymmetry is expected. Also, very young babies will cycle through facial expressions quickly as their body develops and learns to make their muscles do what they want. These fleeting glimpses of asymmetry caused by involuntary movements should not trouble you. You should be more concerned with enduring changes in their face before and after their shots.

Smiling

Notice the location of the sides of their mouth when they smile. Is one side not moving up as far as it had been in a previous test? If there is something wrong, the difference will often be significant enough that you will instantly notice it. Also notice the puffiness of each cheek and the shape of each eye. When they smile properly, their cheeks will puff out as their smile widens, which will cause their eyes to "squinch" closed.

If something has changed, you will notice one side of their face remains flat. The eye on that side of their face will look larger, more round. You may be tempted to think the side with the eye that is more closed has developed a problem, but if they are smiling, their eye should close a bit. It's the other side with the flat cheek and wide open eye during a smile that may have a problem.

Frowning

If you are able to catch your baby frowning or crying, note the curvature of their lips. Again, try and use video so that you can go back and grab a still frame of them when their mouth is at its most protracted state. Both sides should be even. Everyone's lips curve in different ways when they are upset, so I wouldn't obsess over the particular shape of their lips. What you are looking for is asymmetry, particularly asymmetry that developed soon after their shots.

This asymmetry can often be observed as a droopy frown. Lester Holt, the NBC news anchor and Milo Ventimiglia are two famous droopy-mouthed celebrities. You can notice this form of 7th cranial nerve palsy when they are talking.

* * *

Blinking

The 7th cranial nerve is also responsible for opening and closing your eyelids when you blink. There are two things you can look out for with this particular test. One is the resting state of their eyelids. If they are in an active state, and you are sure they are not sleepy, note the resting height of their eyelids. Sometimes a 7th cranial nerve palsy will cause retraction of the eyelids to require more effort, and as a result, their eyelids will rest lower down on their eyes, giving them a look of being constantly sleepy. Again, video them before and after, looking straight at the camera so that you have something to compare to later.

The second blinking test should employ slo-motion video on your phone if you have it. With your baby alert and nowhere near nap time, record their face with the slo-motion video and lightly blow a puff of air on their eyes, making them blink. You may not be able to detect it in real-time, but playing back the slo-motion video should reveal any problems with this part of the 7th cranial nerve. Their blinks should be evenly timed and close fully on both eyes. A problem with this cranial nerve will cause the blinks to appear to happen at different times, as if they are out of sync. What is actually happening is one eyelid cannot close completely and as such begins the retraction phase of the blink before the other. You may be able to see this with a normal speed video, but with the slo-motion video available on some phones, it's very easy to detect.

Unlike some of the other tests mentioned in this chapter, blinking should almost never be asymmetrical. It is an involuntary opening and closing of the eyelid and if for some reason your baby's aren't closing fully on one side, I would mention it to your healthcare provider.

Checking for 3rd, 4th or 6th cranial nerve palsy (Strabismus)

Babies can be difficult to detect strabismus in, both because the bridge of their nose is so wide and because their muscles are just beginning to get coordinated enough for any part of their body to do what they want it to do. As is the case with crooked smiles, the thing we are most concerned with is a sudden change in the alignment of their eyes. Below are a few tips on how you can document and test their eye alignment.

When your baby is looking straight at you, changes in the alignment of their eyes should be relatively easy to spot. Try to take pictures of them, looking straight at you. Again, a video will be easier as you can grab a frame of a squirming baby later, at just the right moment, without worrying about having to time the camera shutter perfectly.

One thing you can do to detect subtle changes in their eye alignment is use the flash on your phone when you take their picture. Put a piece of transparent tape over the LED if you feel it's too bright. The flash is not used to make the image brighter but serves a different purpose—it will show up in the photograph as a distinct white dot in the pupils of your child's eyes and can provide a registration mark for detailed comparison. You may need to zoom into the photo to be able to see it, but in babies with strabismus you might notice the white dot is just inside the pupil on one side while just outside the pupil on the other. A difference between the eyes is not as concerning as detecting a change in their eye positions before and after their shots.

The second technique you can use may require some assistance but will allow you to pick up on other cranial nerve palsies that might go otherwise undetected.

If your child is old enough to understand your commands, ask them to hold their head still, looking straight forward. If you have an infant, you may need someone to grasp the top of their head and hold it still. Make a video of this process so you can compare it with later versions.

With the tip of your finger (or some other object that your baby will fixate on), draw a large circle around the outside of their head, like you're tracing the face of a clock. Draw it just big enough they have to move their eyes significantly to track it. You can ask your younger children to track your finger but little ones may need some encouragement.

Your child's eyes should both track evenly as they move around the circle. If your child has weakness in one of their oculomotor muscles, you will notice that in certain directions (usually the extreme sides or corners) one of their eyes will not be able to move as far as the other. These techniques will allow you to spot subtle potential problems with the cranial nerves that control their eyes.

If you notice that one of your child's eyes deviates inward towards their nose, that is an indication they may have 6th cranial nerve palsy. The 6th cranial nerve serves to enervate the muscle that pulls the eye outward, away from the nose. If it has an issue, the muscles can't pull the eye outward and it tends to turn inwards. Even if at a normal resting position you don't see it, you may notice one eye track outwardly less than the other as their eye follows your finger around the circle.

If you notice that one of your child's eye deviates outward, away from their nose, this may be a sign they've developed a 3rd cranial nerve palsy. The 3rd cranial nerve enervates the muscle that pulls their eye inward towards the nose. When it is not working correctly, the eye tends to drift outward. During the circle exercise, you may notice one of the eyes not pulling inward as far as it should. If this is the case, your child may have a 3rd cranial nerve palsy.

The 3rd cranial nerve pulls your eyes both up and down and as such an imbalance between the two sides may not be as obvious. There are two types of strabismus where one eye is higher or lower than the other. These are very uncommon because the same nerve controls both directions. You may notice as their eyes follow the circle that one eye does not look up or down as far as the others. This could be a sign they have a 3rd cranial nerve palsy.

If you notice one of the eyes moving upwards when it moves in towards the nose, this may be caused by a 4th cranial nerve palsy. This movement is more subtle than the others and can be difficult to discern. If you think about the circle you draw as the face of a clock, you might see your child's left eye shoot upwards as it tries to follow your finger towards the 9 o'clock mark. Conversely, you might notice their right eye shoot upwards as it looks towards their nose as your finger reaches the 3 o'clock mark.

If you spot significant changes in the resting position or motion of your child's eyes soon after their shots, they may have developed cranial nerve palsy in either their 3rd, 4th or 6th cranial nerves.

Checking for hearing-related cranial nerve palsy (7th and 8th)

The 8th cranial nerve is called the vestibulocochlear nerve and transmits sound and motion inputs to the brain. It is responsible for hearing and balance. The 7th cranial nerve, which controls the face, also plays a small but very important role in hearing.

Hearing—7th and 8th cranial nerve palsy tests

For a baby who is not speaking yet, it can be difficult to ascertain whether they may have cranial nerve damage that affects their hearing. This is because cranial nerve damage can make them *more* sensitive to certain noises (not necessarily loud noises). What causes problems? A tiny branch of the 7th cranial nerve, the part that controls the face, also controls the stapedius muscle in your ear, the tiniest muscle in your body. This muscle's purpose is to dampen vibrations on the eardrum, which prevents noises from being too loud. If that muscle is not functioning properly due to a 7th cranial nerve lesion, you might perceive certain sounds extremely loud, to the point you may feel excruciating pain at the most innocent of noises.

It can also make distinguishing human speech from background noise difficult. The occurrence of this phenomenon is nearly impossible to confirm with someone who can't speak. And in a particularly cruel irony, if it occurs early on in life, it can make learning to speak difficult.

Problems with the 8th cranial nerve and hearing are poorly understood, but according to the medical literature appear to cause hypersensitivity in some and poor hearing—perhaps poor sound "cognition"—in others.

How might you at least test for hypersensitivity? The list of possible things that might trigger pain in your child's hearing should they develop a 7th or 8th cranial nerve palsy is endless, and as such makes a before/after style test seem futile. I will describe something you might try if you are willing. It may be helpful to simply keep the objective of this test in mind as you observe your child before and after their vaccines.

Begin taking mental note of things that create specific noises in your home. A dog barking. A vacuum cleaner. An older sibling playing the piano. The washing machine. A door bell. Anything that is a distinct noise you can easily recreate. Again—loud is not the objective. Something specific and reproducible. Take a video of your baby while creating these specific noises. It is unlikely that your baby will react to any of these noises if their hearing is fine. In later tests, create the same noises and see if they react. If you can sense pain on their face with a noise that was formerly benign, they may have developed a problem with their 7th or 8th cranial nerve.

Again, you are unlikely to find that one sound that triggers them before there is a problem—most people would only notice something after many repetitions of the same pattern. A baby suddenly seems very upset or in pain for no apparent reason. Nothing appears to have changed. Eventually, after 10 episodes, you realize that this cry of pain is triggered by the spin cycle on the washing machine.

Motion—8th cranial nerve palsy tests

In addition to hearing, the vestibulocochlear nerve allows your brain to process movement and spatial orientation. Problems with the 8th cranial nerve can be observed in the eyes. Conduct this test the day before their shots, the day after and then the week after.

With your baby laying on their back and at a time when they can be fully engaged with you (not sleepy, fussy, etc.), grasp both sides of their head and gently turn it to the left and right. Their eyes should automatically compensate for this movement and easily track your face even though their head is being rotated.

Then pull their head forward and push it back. Again, their eyes should be able to smoothly track your face even though the positioning of their head is being changed.

If you notice a sudden difference in your baby's ability to track stationary objects with their eyes while their head is moving, it may be a sign they have developed an 8th cranial nerve palsy. If this happens you might notice their eyes jump around as they attempt to center you in their view or possibly a long delay in their ability to focus on you.

A second test you can try is called the Protective Extension test. With your baby facing away from you, grasp them around their torso and hold them in the air. Gently but quickly tilt them forward towards the ground. Their arms should splay out in front of them in a reflexive action to protect themselves from a possible fall. If their 8th cranial nerve is working properly, their vestibular system should detect the sudden tilt and reflexively throw their arms out to prevent injury. A lack of this response may indicate a problem with their 8th cranial nerve.

The results of the Protective Extension test should be taken into consideration alongside the results of the 11th cranial nerve test, as these two cranial nerves work together to provide both the spatial positioning and neck and shoulder support necessary to respond correctly to this action.

9th and 10th cranial nerve palsies

The scope of symptoms caused by 9th and 10th cranial nerve problems is vast and may be difficult to test with specific before and after photographs or videos. Additionally, isolating some problems to the 9th cranial nerve specifically is nearly impossible. Regardless, I will go through a few things you can watch out for should you believe something significant may have changed with your child after their shots.

Although difficult to detect in a baby, a 9th cranial nerve lesion can cause the sound of their voice to change. It may become nasal-sounding, with air tending to flow through their nose rather than their mouth. If you notice this phenomenon, make sure you also scrutinize the 12th cranial nerve tests because if they occur together, it may cause serious speech impairments.

A common issue associated with 9th and/or 10th cranial nerve palsy is a sudden change in eating habits. These nerves work together to coordinate the swallowing mechanism and problems may be noted by an apparent unwillingness to eat or an increase in regurgitated food. Some mothers mistakenly believe their child has suddenly developed an allergy to their own breastmilk after vaccines when in fact their child simply has trouble swallowing due to a 9th or 10th cranial nerve lesion.

A lesion to the 10th cranial nerve can cause many different, seemingly unrelated issues, from behavioral changes to gut issues like constipation or loose stools. It is beyond the scope of this battery of tests to exhaustively describe 10th cranial nerve lesions. If your child has developed a sudden change in sleeping habits, anxiety, gut issues or any other seemingly unexplainable behaviors, look up the function of the vagus nerve and see if their might be some connection. I've found that many changes parents see in their children after vaccination can be attributed to 10th cranial nerve palsies.

Checking for 11th cranial nerve palsy

The *accessory* cranial nerve controls many of your neck muscles. Interestingly, tests for problems with your 11th cranial nerve already exist although healthcare providers have apparently not made the connection that 11th cranial nerve lesions may be the cause. It is my theory that 11th cranial nerve palsy may be the cause of *torticollis* and *head lag*. Torticollis is described as "when your child's head persistently tilts to one side."[241] If you'd like to read more about this phenomenon, please read the chapter on Torticollis.

When the sternocleidomastoid muscle pairs towards the front of your neck and the trapezius muscle pairs on the back of your neck work in tandem, they allow your head to remain straight and upright.

A newborn lacks enough muscle tone in their neck for testing, but if your baby is at least 2 months old, you should be able to conduct this test. You will probably need someone to assist you in capturing these particular tests on video as they will require both hands in assisting your child.

Reminder

As is the case with all of these tests, we are looking for a significant change in behavior in the before/after sequence more than anything else. Every child is different and timing differences between the development of this or that skill should be expected to a degree.

* * *

11th cranial nerve test for 2 to 3 month olds

The day before your baby is due for their shots, lay them on their back, grasp their hands and pull them towards you into a sitting position. You will notice their head lag behind their upper body, but once they are sitting upright (with your hands supporting their torso), they should be able to hold their head straight. It should not collapse forward onto their chest or fall backwards. They will bob and weave a bit as they maintain this position, but in general their head should remain upright.

Most babies will look straight ahead during this maneuver as distributing the weight of their head across both sternocleidomastoid muscles makes it easier. Take note of whether their head falls or twists to one side as you raise them into a sitting position—this may indicate an issue with their 11th cranial nerve.

Then lay them on their stomach and notice the amount of lift they are able to achieve with their head. With some encouragement, you should see them be able to lift their head for a few seconds at a time.

Repeat this sequence of movements a day after they get their shots, then a week after they get their shots. Compare any differences. If you notice a significant change in their ability to hold their head upright, or if you notice their head twisting to one side during the pull-to-sit exercise, they may have developed a lesion on their 11th cranial nerve.

11th cranial nerve test for 4 to 6 month olds

Repeat the same test as described above for your 4 to 6 month old baby before and after their shots. When you do the pull-to-sit exercise, by around 6 months old you shouldn't see any head lag. Their head should stay in line with their trunk as you pull them into the vertical position. It should not twist as they come up, and it should not fall back or forward once they are upright.

As with the other tests, the important thing to note is a difference in behaviors before and after their shots.

12th cranial nerve test

The hypoglossal nerve controls most of the movement of your tongue. After having noticed before/after pictures of children with significant tongue protrusion, I suspect damage to the 12th cranial nerve can actually cause two separate issues common in babies.

12th cranial nerve tests in babies

You don't need to take specific pictures or videos for this test, but within the before/after sequence you are going to conduct around each time your child gets their shots, take note of their tongue. When they are actively engaged with you, and are not eating or attempting to put something in their mouth, notice their tongue. Does it retract fully? Is it sometimes hidden from view, even when their mouth is open? Or does it hang outside their mouth, slightly protruding beyond their lips, even with their mouth apparently closed.

Similarly, if you are breastfeeding your child, take note of their ability to latch before and after they receive their shots. I've heard stories from lactation consultants who have noticed many infants lose their ability to latch after vaccines, something you might attribute to them losing mobility in their tongue.

With either of these tests—tongue protrusion or latching ability—if you notice a significant change after your child receives their shots, they may have developed a 12th cranial nerve palsy—something that can cause paralysis in their tongue. You may want to look into a healthy alternative to vaccines.

12th cranial nerve tests in children

I believe that lesions on the 12th cranial nerve may be responsible for some speech delays due to difficulty forming the correct tongue shapes for different speech phonemes. If you'd like to monitor your child closely, there are few tests you can do to spot if something has happened to their 12th cranial nerve.

Once your child is old enough to follow your commands, and is at least partially vocal, record this sequence of sounds/words the day before their shots, then the day and week after.

1) "Gosh." Try and get them to make a "Guh" sound. This sound requires the back 1/3 of the tongue to move up and temporarily stop the air from flowing. Record them saying "gosh." Note their ability to create this sound properly.

2) "Sss." Try to get them to make an "s" sound. This sound requires air to flow through a small gap in the middle of the tip of the tongue. If they lack control of their tongue, it will often not be able to form this specific shape and air will flow over the sides instead, creating what is known as a *lateral lisp*.

3) "Off." Try to get them to make an "f" sound. This sound requires nothing from the tongue other than staying out of the way. If they are unable to make the "f" sound, they may lack enough control of their tongue to pull it down.

4) "Ell." Try to get them to make an "l" sound. This tricky sound requires some coordination from the tip of the tongue and can be difficult without full control.

5) "Juice." Try to get them to make a "j" sound. This sound is another tricky shape to make with your tongue and the inability to make this sound can indicate partial tongue paralysis.

6) "Dad." Try to get them to make a "d" sound. This sound requires coordination from the tongue—the back part of the tongue must stay lower in the mouth, curving up towards the tip as it depresses against the back of the teeth.

* * *

Go through this battery of sounds before and after your child's shots, or as soon as they are able. Every child is different and the age at which they are able to make these tongue-specific sounds will vary. We are more concerned with a sudden inability to make these sounds where they had once been able to. If your child was able to make these sounds in a previous video, and now cannot, they may have developed a 12th cranial nerve palsy causing partial paralysis of their tongue.

Conclusion

This is a lot of tests and may seem like a lot to worry about over nothing. However, many parents are convinced their child changed in some way after their vaccines but aren't quite able to put their finger on it. When they bring up these concerns to their pediatricians, they are often left to vaguely describe what seemed to be a sudden change in their child with no proof that something actually happened.

Unfortunately, when it comes to vaccines, pediatricians are too quick to shift the blame to coincidence or an overly-concerned mother. These tests will arm you with both the confidence that something did change, and give you the ability to approach your pediatrician with indisputable proof of this change. With these videos or pictures on your phone, your next visit to the pediatrician should allow them to be more focused on healing and treatment rather than doubting your concerns.

EPILOGUE

No. XXVII. Partial Paralysis.

"A healthy male child, four months old, of a plethoric habit, was very restless during the night of the 11th of August; a dose of calomel and scammony had been given him the day before, and the mother supposed the restlessness was owing to this circumstance. She observed, however, that when he cried, his face was drawn forcibly to the left side. 12th. The aperient[i] was repeated 13th. On a careful examination there is nothing remarkable behind the ear or about the angle of the jaw... With the exception of the eye, the features on this side of the face of this lively laughing little fellow are quite without expression."[242]

Charles Bell would go on to describe many more cases of people, even babies, that would develop this strange affliction few had ever seen—one half of their face would stop working. It's rare you will see an account where medicinal metals of the day weren't administered

---

i. *Any drug used to relieve constipation.*

directly before the paralysis appeared, and for that reason, I'm fairly certain that mercury was causing the asymmetrical facial weakness that would come to be known as Bell's Palsy,

What of today? The lead pipes that poisoned our water supplies are long gone and mercury is seldom administered. But we have a new metal, one that might be more insidious than either of them. Aluminum is everywhere in trace amounts and is in our vaccines in potentially deadly quantities. The enormous volume of mercury it took to temporarily injure a 7th cranial nerve nuclei in the early 1800s has been replaced with a couple hundred micrograms of aluminum injected into the body and delivered to the worst of all places with pinpoint accuracy. Today's Bell's Palsy patients often receive their paralysis years after the metal has been injected—a surprise gift inside the white blood cells of the immune system, transported to the brain due to some otherwise trivial infection.

The great scientific minds of Charles Bell's day could not piece together the effects of metal and medicine—even though it was sitting right there in front of them, visible in nearly every report they made. It's not hard to imagine how—with possibly a years-long disconnect between cause and effect—the best doctors and researchers of today have been unable to make the connection between vaccines and aluminum.

You may be wondering where you fit in to this puzzle if the specifics of your disorder weren't mentioned. This book covers a few of the more common man-made diseases, but there were many others I had to skip such as ALS, Sepsis, SIDS, and some of the Ehlers-Danlos syndromes. Quite a few cancers appear to be directly correlated with man—that is no surprise, but it runs deeper than you might imagine. Environmental exposure to metals have long been associated with lung, lymphoma and pancreatic cancer, but the chronic inflammation many experience may also be a trigger.

Even the errant cell differentiation process observed in leukemia has been linked to problems caused by elevated vitamin D1,25 levels—a common sign of a body struggling to fight off intracellular bacterial infections. Cancer appears to have existed in some form throughout much of recorded history, but one can only wonder to what extent. Hopefully, if the illness you are experiencing was not mentioned, you are still able to piece together what may be causing your suffering. These diseases might just be different symptoms of the same phenomenon after all—a combination of metal toxicity and the chronic inflammation they help create.

When it comes to any flavor of modern disease, it would appear that humanity is content to ask the same two questions: What are the genetic defects that caused this? When can we expect a cure? One might think that if any of these diseases were determined to have a human cause, there would be rejoicing in the streets. A man-made cause should theoretically be reversible, which would make the disease preventable. But for some reason, we always look the other way when a human-centered role is implied.

We are all desperate for a cure, healing or the knowledge that could allow prevention. Why is it so many are reluctant to admit human complicity in these diseases? Could they be uncomfortable with their potential role in causing the very problem they purport to stop? Or like "Red" in Shawshank Redemption, might they be uncomfortable with thoughts of life "on the outside," once their skills are no longer needed?

A curious phenomenon regarding scientific discovery was eloquently stated in *Age of Autism*:

> *"Whenever germs are discovered to be an essential part of a disease process, we typically attribute causation solely to the germ. We generally accept that the measles virus "causes" SSPE and the poliovirus "causes" paralysis even though we don't know why the condition turns pathogenic in some cases and not in*

others. By contrast, in the case of conditions where an environmental exposure is identified as a cause of a disease, instead of linking the exposure with the disease, the most frequent response is to remove the disease label from the case."[243]

Might our reluctance to call the modern illnesses "disease" be a clear indication as to the middle-ground we occupy? A gnawing, unspoken sense that perhaps even if the environmental cause is not identified, the "woods in which it lives" is known?

For all of the progress that humans have achieved in the last two hundred years, we have at least set our cause back that far. When measured in terms of the "rattle and hum" of all the machinery we've created to monitor our progress, it would appear we have been an unbridled success. Carefully chosen measurements of health can also assure us that our efforts have moved the cause of humanity in a positive direction. Upon a more parsimonious inspection, cracks in the veneer appear, and the metrics by which we congratulate ourselves every minute of every day lose the sparkle they once had.

Humans can be selfish beings, but I believe above all they are mostly compassionate. The same compassion that can provide decades of self-sacrifice in caring for a sick loved one or searching for answers will make facing the reality of their suffering difficult.

The effects of the last two hundred years of metals, microbes and medicine are visible around us. The bodies and minds of all those wrecked from mercuric medicine and arsenical solutions in the 1800s are not even ghosts to us anymore. But we have our own examples through which we should draw inspiration—from the caregivers of struggling Alzheimer's patients to the tireless efforts of parents and their autistic children. From the silent suffering of those with Crohn's, rheumatoid arthritis and fibromyalgia, to the subtle crooked smiles and misaligned eyes that seem to be everywhere. Most of us have been caught up in this story in some way, as a parent or patient. All of us have witnessed what's happened.

With a healthy dose of humility, and a perhaps a little bit of luck, the truth will emerge. Whether this year or the next, it will surface. If the hypotheses put forward in this book are true, then as horrible as they may be, perhaps we can begin to put the finishing touches on this chapter of metal and medicine— then begin again.

NOTES

1. Science Buddies, "Side-Dominant Science: Are You Left- or Right-Sided?", www.scientificamerican.com/article/bring-science-home-dominant-side/
2. Pichot M.D., Amédée, Life and Labours of Sir Charles Bell (London, Richard Bentley), 1860, p. 24.
3. Pichot M.D., Amédée, Life and Labours of Sir Charles Bell (London, Richard Bentley), 1860, p. viii.
4. Bell, Sir Charles, "The nervous system of the human body : embracing the papers delivered to the Royal Society on the subject of the nerves" (Washington : Stereotyped by D. Green, for the Register and Library of Medical and Chirurgical Science, 1833), p. 13.
5. Bell, Sir Charles, "The Anatomy and Philosophy of Expression as Connected with the Fine Arts" (London, John Murray, 1844), p. 21.
6. Mohammad M. Sajadi et. al, "The history of facial palsy and spasm", Neurology (Jul 2011), 77 (2) 174-178
7. Fuller G, Morgan C, "Bell's palsy syndrome: mimics and chameleons", *Practical Neurology* 2016;16:439-444.
8. Farroni T, Menon E, Rigato S, Johnson MH. The perception of facial expressions in newborns. The European Journal of Developmental Psychology. 2007;4(1):2-13. doi:10.1080/17405620601046832.
9. *Bell, Sir Charles, "The nervous system of the human body : embracing the papers delivered to the Royal Society on the subject of the nerves" (Washington : Stereotyped by D. Green, for the Register and Library of Medical and Chirurgical Science, 1833), p. 132.*
10. *Ibid, p. 141-142.*
11. Steckling, Nadine et al. "Disease Profile and Health-Related Quality of Life (HRQoL) Using the EuroQol (EQ-5D + C) Questionnaire for Chronic Metallic Mercury Vapor Intoxication." *Health and Quality of Life Outcomes* 13 (2015): 196. *PMC*. Web. 19 Dec. 2017, https://www.ncbi.nlm.nih.gov/pmc/

articles/PMC4675011/#CR37

12. Johnson HR, Koumides O. Unusual case of mercury poisoning. *British Medical Journal*. 1967;1(5536): 340-341, ncbi.nlm.nih.gov/pmc/articles/PMC1840764/?page=1

13. "Diet-related mercury poisoning resulting in visual loss", Saldana et. al, Br J Ophthalmol. 2006 Nov; 90(11): 1432–1434, https://www.ncbi.nlm.nih.gov/pmc/articles/PMC1857490/

14. *Bell, Sir Charles, "The nervous system of the human body : embracing the papers delivered to the Royal Society on the subject of the nerves" (Washington : Stereotyped by D. Green, for the Register and Library of Medical and Chirurgical Science, 1833), p. 147-148.*

15. https://en.wikipedia.org/wiki/Chinese_alchemical_elixir_poisoning

16. "Positional Plagiocephaly and Sleep Positioning: An Update to the Joint Statement on Sudden Infant Death Syndrome." Paediatrics & Child Health 6.10 (2001): 788–789. Print, https://www.ncbi.nlm.nih.gov/pmc/articles/PMC2805995/

17. Stellwagen L, Hubbard E, Chambers C, et al Torticollis, facial asymmetry and plagiocephaly in normal newborns Archives of Disease in Childhood 2008;93:827-831.

18. Lee, KyeongSoo, EunJung Chung, and Byoung-Hee Lee. "A Comparison of Outcomes of Asymmetry in Infants with Congenital Muscular Torticollis according to Age upon Starting Treatment." Journal of Physical Therapy Science 29.3 (2017): 543–547. PMC. Web. 20 Dec. 2017.

19. Long-Term Developmental Outcomes in Patients With Deformational Plagiocephaly, Robert I. Miller, Sterling K. Clarren, Pediatrics Feb 2000, 105 (2) e26; DOI: 10.1542/peds.105.2.e26

20. Kekunnaya, Ramesh, and Sherwin J Isenberg. "Effect of Strabismus Surgery on Torticollis Caused by Congenital Superior Oblique Palsy in Young Children." Indian Journal of Ophthalmology 62.3 (2014): 322–326. PMC. Web. 20 Dec. 2017.

21. *Bell, Sir Charles, "The nervous system of the human body : embracing the papers delivered to the Royal Society on the subject of the nerves" (Washington : Stereotyped by D. Green, for the Register and Library of Medical and Chirurgical Science, 1833), p. 156-159.*

22. Haslam, Jessica Charlotte, "Deadly décor: a short history of arsenic poisoning in the nineteenth century", *Vol 21, Issue 1, Res Medica: Journal of the Royal Medical Society* (Edinburgh, 2013), p. 79.

23. Bell, Sir Charles, "The nervous system of the human body : embracing the papers delivered to the Royal Society on the subject of the nerves" (Washington : Stereotyped by D. Green, for the Register and Library of Medical and Chirurgical Science, 1833), p. 159.

24. Ibid.

25. Zablotsky B, Black LI, Blumberg SJ. Estimated prevalence of children with diagnosed developmental disabilities in the United States, 2014–2016. NCHS Data Brief, no 291. Hyattsville, MD: National Center for Health Statistics. 2017.

26. Flanagan, J. E., Landa, R., Bhat, A., & Bauman, M. (2012). Head lag in infants at risk for autism: A preliminary study. American Journal of Occupational Therapy, 66(5), 577-585. DOI: 10.5014/ajot.2012.004192

27. DeMyer WE, Zeman W, Palmer CG. The face predicts the brain: diagnostic significance of median facial anomalies for holoprosencephaly (arhinencephaly). Pediatrics 1964; 34: 256–263.

28. Lyons-Weiler , James. The Environmental and Genetic Causes of Autism . Skyhorse Publishing. Kindle Edition, loc. 142

29. Ibid.

30. Hammond P, Forster-Gibson C, Chudley AE, Allanson JE, Hutton TJ, Farrell SA, et al. Face-brain asymmetry in autism spectrum disorders. Mol Psychiatry. 2008;13:614–623. doi: 10.1038/mp.2008.18.

31. *Hammond P, Forster-Gibson C, Chudley AE, Allanson JE, Hutton TJ, Farrell SA, et al. Face-brain asymmetry in autism spectrum disorders. Mol Psychiatry. 2008;13:614–623. doi: 10.1038/mp.2008.18.*

32. George M. Beard, "A Practical Treatise on Nervous Exhaustion (Neurasthenia)— Its Symptoms, Nature, Sequences, Treatment" (New York: William Wood & Co., 1880), 9.

33. *"The Treatment of Neurasthenia," Gilbert Ballet, 3rd Edition, 1905, p. xxvi.*

34. Evengård, B., Schacterle, R. S. and Komaroff , A. L. (1999), Chronic fatigue syndrome: new insights and old ignorance. Journal of Internal Medicine, 246: 455–469. doi:10.1046/j.1365-2796.1999.00513.x

35. Jamieson, Hurry, "The vicious circles of neurasthenia, and their treatment," London: Churchill, 1915

36. Beard, George, "Neurasthenia, or nervous exhaustion", Boston Med Surg J 1869; 80:217-221 April 29, 1869, DOI: 10.1056/NEJM186904290801301

37. Wigglesworth Jr. M.D., Edward, "Subcutaneous Injection of Corrosive Sublimate in Syphilis," Boston

Med Surg J 1869; 81:49-51August 26, 1869, DOI: 10.1056/NEJM186908260810401

38. Taylor, Ruth E., "Death of neurasthenia and its psychological reincarnation," The British Journal of Psychiatry Dec 2001, 179 (6) 550-557; DOI: 10.1192/bjp.179.6.550

39. https://www.fda.gov/MedicalDevices/ProductsandMedicalProcedures/DentalProducts/DentalAmalgam/ucm171094.htm

40. Taylor, Ruth E., "Death of neurasthenia and its psychological reincarnation," The British Journal of Psychiatry Dec 2001, 179 (6) 550-557; DOI: 10.1192/bjp.179.6.550

41. Bloom WL, Flinchum D. "Osteomalacia with pseudofractures caused by the ingestion of aluminium hydroxide," JAMA 1960;174:1327–30.

42. Betts, Dr. Charles T., "The Aluminum Octopus," Research Publishing Company, Toledo, Ohio, p. 1.

43. De Gregorio, Ennio, Elena Caproni, and Jeffrey B. Ulmer. "Vaccine Adjuvants: Mode of Action." Frontiers in Immunology 4 (2013): 214. PMC. Web. 20 Dec. 2017.

44. *Döllken, v. Ueber die wirkung des aluminiums mit besonderer beriicksichtigung der durch das aluminium verursachten lasionen im centralnervensystem. Archiv. Exp. Path. Pharmaco., 1898, 40, 98-120, https://link.springer.com/article/10.1007%2FBF01931503*

45. Wilson, Rhonda H. et al. "Allergic Sensitization through the Airway Primes Th17-Dependent Neutrophilia and Airway Hyperresponsiveness." American Journal of Respiratory and Critical Care Medicine 180.8 (2009): 720–730. PMC. Web. 20 Dec. 2017.

46. "Proceedings of the Physiological Society, 23-24 February 1968, Institute of Psychiatry Meeting: Demonstrations." *The Journal of Physiology* 196.Suppl (1968): 93P–109P. Print.

47. Gherardi, Romain K., and François-Jérôme Authier. "Macrophagic Myofasciitis: Characterization and Pathophysiology." Lupus 21.2 (2012): 184–189. PMC. Web. 30 Dec. 2017.

48. Atypical presentation of macrophagic myofasciitis 10 years post vaccination Ryan, Aisling M. et al. Neuromuscular Disorders , Volume 16 , Issue 12 , 867 - 869

49. Luján, L., Pérez, M., Salazar, E. et al. "Autoimmune/autoinflammatory syndrome induced by adjuvants (ASIA syndrome) in commercial sheep," Immunol Res (2013) 56: 317. https://doi.org/10.1007/s12026-013-8404-0

50. This study has not been published at this time. The lead author is Luján, L.

51. Guillemette Crépeaux, Housam Eidi, Marie-Odile David, Yasmine Baba-Amer, Eleni Tzavara, Bruno Giros, François-Jérôme Authier, Christopher Exley, Christopher A. Shaw, Josette Cadusseau, Romain K. Gherardi, "Non-linear dose-response of aluminium hydroxide adjuvant particles: Selective low dose neurotoxicity, In Toxicology," Volume 375, 2017, Pages 48-57, ISSN 0300-483X, https://doi.org/10.1016/j.tox.2016.11.018. (http://www.sciencedirect.com/science/article/pii/S0300483X16303043)

52. Guillemette Crépeaux, Housam Eidi, Marie-Odile David, Eleni Tzavara, Bruno Giros, Christopher Exley, Patrick A. Curmi, Christopher A. Shaw, Romain K. Gherardi, Josette Cadusseau, Highly delayed systemic translocation of aluminum-based adjuvant in CD1 mice following intramuscular injections, Journal of Inorganic Biochemistry, Volume 152, 2015, Pages 199-205, ISSN 0162-0134, https://doi.org/10.1016/j.jinorgbio.2015.07.004.

53. Anne-Cécile Rimaniol, Gabriel Gras, François Verdier, Francis Capel, Vladimir B Grigoriev, Fabrice Porcheray, Elisabeth Sauzeat, Jean-Guy Fournier, Pascal Clayette, Claire-Anne Siegrist, Dominique Dormont, "Aluminum hydroxide adjuvant induces macrophage differentiation towards a specialized antigen-presenting cell type," In Vaccine, Volume 22, Issues 23–24, 2004, Pages 3127-3135, ISSN 0264-410X, https://doi.org/10.1016/j.vaccine.2004.01.061.

54. Charlotte D'Mello, Tai Le, Mark G. Swain, "Cerebral Microglia Recruit Monocytes into the Brain in Response to Tumor Necrosis Factorα Signaling during Peripheral Organ Inflammation," Journal of Neuroscience 18 February 2009, 29 (7) 2089-2102; DOI: 10.1523/JNEUROSCI.3567-08.2009

55. Woo, Im-Sun, In-Koo Rhee, and Heui-Dong Park. "Differential Damage in Bacterial Cells by Microwave Radiation on the Basis of Cell Wall Structure." Applied and Environmental Microbiology 66.5 (2000): 2243–2247. Print.

56. Pizarro-Cerdá, Javier et al., "Bacterial Adhesion and Entry into Host Cells," Cell, Volume 124, Issue 4 , 715 - 72

57. Renn, C.N., Straff, W., Dorfmüller, A., Al-Masaoudi, T., Merk, H.F. and Sachs, B., "Amoxicillin-induced exanthema in young adults with infectious mononucleosis: demonstration of drug-specific lymphocyte

reactivity," (2002), British Journal of Dermatology, 147: 1166–1170. doi:10.1046/j.1365-2133.2002.05021.x

58. *LERNER, A. (2007), Aluminum Is a Potential Environmental Factor for Crohn's Disease Induction. Annals of the New York Academy of Sciences, 1107: 329–345. doi:10.1196/annals.1381.035.*

59. Saçan, M.T., Oztay, F. & Bolkent, S. Biol Trace Elem Res (2007) 120: 264. https://doi.org/10.1007/s12011-007-8016-4.

60. David L Jones, Leon V Kochian, Aluminum interaction with plasma membrane lipids and enzyme metal binding sites and its potential role in Al cytotoxicity, In FEBS Letters, Volume 400, Issue 1, 1997, Pages 51-57, ISSN 0014-5793, https://doi.org/10.1016/S0014-5793(96)01319-1.

61. Caverly, Charles S., "Infantile Paralysis in Vermont," State Department of Public Health, 1924, p. 28.

62. Minshal C , Nadal J , Exley C ((2014)) Aluminium in human sweat. J Trace Elem Med Biol 28:, 87–88.

63. "The influence of scrotal heating prior to vasectomy on sperm granuloma formation and testicular activity," Subhas, T. et al. Contraception, Volume 21, Issue 2, 175-181.

64. Bennett RG, Heimann DG, Tuma DJ. Relaxin Reduces Fibrosis in Models of Progressive and Established Hepatic Fibrosis. Annals of the New York Academy of Sciences. 2009;1160:348-349. doi: 10.1111/j.1749-6632.2008.03783.x.

65. D A Drossman, "Presidential address: Gastrointestinal illness and the biopsychosocial model," Psychosomatic Medicine. 60(3):258-67, MAY 1998, PMID: 9625212

66. J.G.Goldberg, *Pyschotherapeutic Treatment of Cancer Patients,* p. 45.

67. Moffett A., Loke C., "Immunology of placentation in eutherian mammals," Nat. Rev. Immunol. 2006;6:584–594. doi: 10.1038/nri1897.

68. Mor G, Cardenas I. The Immune System in Pregnancy: A Unique Complexity. American journal of reproductive immunology (New York, NY: 1989). 2010;63(6):425-433. doi:10.1111/j.1600-0897.2010.00836.x.

69. Collins MK, Tay C-S, Erlebacher A. Dendritic cell entrapment within the pregnant uterus inhibits immune surveillance of the maternal/fetal interface in mice. The Journal of Clinical Investigation. 2009;119(7):2062-2073. doi:10.1172/JCI38714.

70. Sidney B. Lang, Andrew A. Marino, Garry Berkovic, Marjorie Fowler, Kenneth D. Abreo, Piezoelectricity in the human pineal gland, In Bioelectrochemistry and Bioenergetics, Volume 41, Issue 2, 1996, Pages 191-195, ISSN 0302-4598, https://doi.org/10.1016/S0302-4598(96)05147-1.

71. *Bell, Sir Charles, The nervous system of the human body : embracing the papers delivered to the Royal Society on the subject of the nerves (Washington : Stereotyped by D. Green, for the Register and Library of Medical and Chirurgical Science, 1833), p. 50*

72. "Macrophagic myofasciitis lesions assess long-term persistence of vaccine-derived aluminium hydroxide in muscle.", Gherardi et. al, https://www.ncbi.nlm.nih.gov/pubmed/11522584

73. https://www.cdc.gov/vaccinesafety/concerns/adjuvants.html

74. "Virtual dissection: a lesson from the 18th century", Lukić, Ivan Krešimir et al, The Lancet , Volume 362, Issue 9401, 2110-2113

75. Ibid.

76. Ibid.

77. "They'll have to rewrite the Textbooks", Barney, Josh, March 31, 2016, https://news.virginia.edu/illimitable/discovery/theyll-have-rewrite-textbooks

78. "Surprise! Scientists Discover the Human Brain Has a Lymphatic System", Berman, Robby, Big Think, October 12, 2017, http://bigthink.com/robby-berman/surprise-scientists-discover-the-human-brain-has-a-lymphatic-system

79. Thomas R, Sanders S, Doust J, Beller E, Glasziou P, "Prevalence of attention-deficit/hyperactivity disorder: a systematic review and meta-analysis," Pediatrics. 2015 Apr; 135(4):e994-1001.

80. Gary Aston-Jones, Janusz Rajkowski, Jonathan Cohen, Role of locus coeruleus in attention and behavioral flexibility, Biological Psychiatry, Volume 46, Issue 9, 1999, Pages 1309-1320, ISSN 0006-3223, https://doi.org/10.1016/S0006-3223(99)00140-7.

81. P.J. Barlow, A pilot study on the metal levels in the hair of hyperactive children, Medical Hypotheses, Volume 11, Issue 3, 1983, Pages 309-318, ISSN 0306-9877, https://doi.org/10.1016/0306-9877(83)90094-4.

82. *Mehler MF, Purpura DP. Autism, fever, epigenetics and the locus coeruleus. Brain research reviews. 2009;59(2):388-392. doi:10.1016/j.brainresrev.2008.11.001.*

83. Almeida, M. C., Steiner, A. A., Coimbra, N. C. and Branco, L. G. S. (2004), Thermoeffector neuronal pathways in fever: a study in rats showing a new role of the locus coeruleus. The Journal of Physiology, 558:

283–294. doi:10.1113/jphysiol.2004.066654.

84. Foss-Feig, Jennifer, et. al, "A Substantial and Unexpected Enhancement of Motion Perception in Autism", Journal of Neuroscience 8 May 2013, 33 (19) 8243-8249; DOI: 10.1523/JNEUROSCI. 1608-12.2013

85. Hill, Jennifer W. "PVN Pathways Controlling Energy Homeostasis." Indian Journal of Endocrinology and Metabolism 16.Suppl 3 (2012): S627–S636. PMC. Web. 27 Dec. 2017.

86. *Porges, Stephen W.. The Pocket Guide to the Polyvagal Theory: The Transformative Power of Feeling Safe (Norton Series on Interpersonal Neurobiology) (Kindle Locations 2203-2204). W. W. Norton & Company. Kindle Edition.*

87. Theologides A., "Anorexia-producing intermediary metabolites," Am J Clin Nutr. 1976 May;29(5): 552-8.

88. Ida A.K. Nilsson, Charlotte Lindfors, Martin Schalling, Tomas Hökfelt, Jeanette E. Johansen, "Chapter Two - Anorexia and Hypothalamic Degeneration, Editor(s): Gerald Litwack, Vitamins & Hormones," Academic Press, Volume 92, 2013, Pages 27-60, ISSN 0083-6729, ISBN 9780124104730, https://doi.org/ 10.1016/B978-0-12-410473-0.00002-7.

89. Mattson, Mark P. "Superior Pattern Processing Is the Essence of the Evolved Human Brain." Frontiers in Neuroscience 8 (2014): 265. PMC. Web. 31 Dec. 2017.

90. Chandler, Rebecca E. et al. "Current Safety Concerns with Human Papillomavirus Vaccine: A Cluster Analysis of Reports in VigiBase®." Drug Safety 40.1 (2017): 81–90. PMC. Web. 30 Dec. 2017.

91. Yates, Bill J, Philip S. Bolton, and Vaughan G. Macefield. "Vestibulo-Sympathetic Responses." Comprehensive Physiology 4.2 (2014): 851–887. PMC. Web. 30 Dec. 2017.

92. *Turnbull, Alexander, "A Treatise on Painful and Nervous Diseases And on a New Mode of Treatment for Diseases of the Eye and Ear", Third Edition, London, 1837, p. 10-11.*

93. *Ibid., p. 12-13.*

94. *Ibid., p. 13-14.*

95. "Autism Spectrum Disorder," Diagnostic and Statistical Manual of Mental Disorders, Fifth Edition, 299.00 (F84.0)

96. *Bell, Sir Charles, "The nervous system of the human body : embracing the papers delivered to the Royal Society on the subject of the nerves" (Washington : Stereotyped by D. Green, for the Register and Library of Medical and Chirurgical Science, 1833), p. 155.*

97. Carson, T. B., et. al. (2017), Vestibulo-ocular reflex function in children with high-functioning autism spectrum disorders. Autism Research, 10: 251–266. doi:10.1002/aur.1642

98. O'Nions, Elizabeth, et. al, "How do Parents Manage Irritability, Challenging Behaviour, Non-Compliance and Anxiety in Children with Autism Spectrum Disorders? A Meta-Synthesis", Journal of Autism and Developmental Disorders, December 8, 2017, https://doi.org/10.1007/s10803-017-3361-4

99. Foss-Feig, Jennifer, et. al, "A Substantial and Unexpected Enhancement of Motion Perception in Autism", Journal of Neuroscience 8 May 2013, 33 (19) 8243-8249; DOI: 10.1523/JNEUROSCI. 1608-12.2013

100. Masataka, Nobuo. "Neurodiversity, Giftedness, and Aesthetic Perceptual Judgment of Music in Children with Autism." Frontiers in Psychology 8 (2017): 1595. PMC. Web. 22 Dec. 2017.

101. Handley, J.B., "Did British Scientists just solve the Autism Puzzle?", Dec. 8, 2017, https://medium.com/ @jbhandley/did-british-scientists-just-solve-the-autism-puzzle-5a7eacc77415

102. Pavlov, Valentin A., and Kevin J. Tracey. "The Vagus Nerve and the Inflammatory Reflex—linking Immunity and Metabolism." Nature reviews. Endocrinology 8.12 (2012): 743–754. PMC. Web. 27 Dec. 2017.

103. Ammori J, Zhang W, Li J, et al. "of intestinal inflammation on neuronal survival and function in the dorsal motor nucleus of the vagus." Surgery. 2009;144:149-158.

104. Assen LM, Ran I, Pittman QJ, et al. Central autonomic activation in TNBS-induced colitis. Gastroenterology. 2003;124(4)(Suppl 1):A116.

105. D'Mello, Charlotte, Le, Tai, Swain, Mark G., "Cerebral Microglia Recruit Monocytes into the Brain in Response to Tumor Necrosis Factorα Signaling during Peripheral Organ Inflammation," Journal of Neuroscience 18 February 2009, 29 (7) 2089-2102; DOI: 10.1523/JNEUROSCI.3567-08.2009

106. Tracey, Kevin J. "Reflex Control of Immunity." Nature reviews. Immunology 9.6 (2009): 418–428. PMC. Web. 27 Dec. 2017.

107. Andersson, Ulf, and Kevin J. Tracey. "Reflex Principles of Immunological Homeostasis." Annual

review of immunology 30 (2012): 313–335. PMC. Web. 27 Dec. 2017.

108. *Alexander Stewart, Captain; Stewart, Cameron; Stewart, Alexander. A Very Unimportant Officer (Kindle Locations 317-319). Hodder & Stoughton. Kindle Edition.*

109. Mitchie H. The venereal diseases. In: Ireland M, ed. The Medical Department of the US Army in the world war. Washington, DC: GPO, 1928: 263–310.

110. Turner, William Aldren, "CASES OF NERVOUS AND MENTAL SHOCK OBSERVED IN THE BASE HOSPITALS OF FRANCE", Br Med J. 1915 May 15; 1(2837): 833–835.

111. *Charles S. Myers, "A Contribution to the Study of Shell Shock," The Lancet, February 13, 1915, p. 316*

112. *Elliott, T. R. "'TRANSIENT PARAPLEGIA FROM SHELL EXPLOSIONS.'" British Medical Journal 2.2815 (1914): 1005–1006. Print.*

113. Alexander Stewart, Captain; Stewart, Cameron; Stewart, Alexander. A Very Unimportant Officer (Kindle Location 1652). Hodder & Stoughton. Kindle Edition.

114. S. Levine and H. Ursin, "What is Stress?" in S. Levine and H. Ursin, eds., Psychobiology of Stress (New York: Academic Press), 17.

115. Wakefield, Andrew J., Stott, Carol, "Autism—an epicenter in the brain stem?" The Autism File, Issue 37, 2010, p. 120-129.

116. Porges, Stephen W.. The Pocket Guide to the Polyvagal Theory: The Transformative Power of Feeling Safe (Norton Series on Interpersonal Neurobiology) (Kindle Location 211). W. W. Norton & Company. Kindle Edition.

117. Sanders, B., and M. Gray. 1997. Early environmental influences can attenuate the blood pressure response to acute stress in borderline hypertensive rats. Physiology and Behavior. 61: 749– 54.

118. Taylor, Shelley E.. The Tending Instinct: Women, Men, and the Biology of Nurturing (Kindle Locations 242-243). Henry Holt and Co.. Kindle Edition.

119. Ibid. (Kindle Locations 294-295).

120. *Ibid. (Kindle Locations 50-52).*

121. Kendrick, K. M., E. B. Keverne, and B. A. Baldwin. 1987. Intracerebroventricular oxytocin stimulates maternal behaviour in the sheep. Neuroendocrinology. 46: 56– 61.

122. *Taylor, Shelley E.. The Tending Instinct: Women, Men, and the Biology of Nurturing (Kindle Locations 400-402). Henry Holt and Co.. Kindle Edition.*

123. *Bostock, John, "Case of a Periodical Affection of the Eyes and Chest," Presented to the Royal Medico-Chirurgical Society of London, 1819, p. 165*

124. *Bostock, John, "Of Catarrhus Æstivus, or Summer Catarrh" Presented to the Royal Medico-Chirurgical Society of London, April 22, 1828, p. 438*

125. *Bostock, John, "Of Catarrhus Æstivus, or Summer Catarrh" Presented to the Royal Medico-Chirurgical Society of London, April 22, 1828, p. 440*

126. E. W. Goodall, "A Clinical Address on Serum Sickness," The Lancet (March 2, 1918), and the Lancet (March 9, 1918).

127. George W. Gray, "Allergy, protection gone wild," Harper's Magazine rerun in the Milwaukee Journal (Sat., Jan. 1, 1939).

128. Exley, Christopher. "Aluminium Adjuvants and Adverse Events in Sub-Cutaneous Allergy Immunotherapy." Allergy, Asthma, and Clinical Immunology: Official Journal of the Canadian Society of Allergy and Clinical Immunology 10.1 (2014): 4. PMC. Web. 27 Dec. 2017.

129. Brunner, R., Wallmann, J., Szalai, K., Karagiannis, P., Kopp, T., Scheiner, O., Jensen-Jarolim, E. and Pali-Schöll, I. (2007), The impact of aluminium in acid-suppressing drugs on the immune response of BALB/c mice. Clinical & Experimental Allergy, 37: 1566–1573. doi:10.1111/j.1365-2222.2007.02813.x

130. Wilson, Rhonda H. et al. "Allergic Sensitization through the Airway Primes Th17-Dependent Neutrophilia and Airway Hyperresponsiveness." American Journal of Respiratory and Critical Care Medicine 180.8 (2009): 720–730. PMC. Web. 28 Dec. 2017.

131. Mishra, Amarjit et al. "Dendritic Cells Induce Th2-Mediated Airway Inflammatory Responses to House Dust Mite via DNA-Dependent Protein Kinase." Nature communications 6 (2015): 6224. PMC. Web. 28 Dec. 2017.

132. A Desjardins , J P Bergeron , H Ghezzo , A Cartier , and J L Malo, "Aluminium potroom asthma confirmed by monitoring of forced expiratory volume in one second," Am J Respir Crit Care Med. 1994 Dec;150(6 Pt 1):1714-7.

133. Vaughan, Warren T., Strange Malady, the Story of Allergy, Doubleday, Doran & Co; First Edition

edition (1941)

134. Hildick-Smith, Gavin , et. al, Penicillin Regimens In Pediatric Practice, Pediatrics Jan 1950, 5 (1) 97-113;

135. *Khodoun, Marat et al. "Peanuts Can Contribute to Anaphylactic Shock by Activating Complement." The Journal of allergy and clinical immunology 123.2 (2009): 342–351. PMC. Web. 28 Dec. 2017.*

136. Smith, K. N., "What's in the Smallpox Vaccine?" Forbes Science, Oct. 11, 2017, https://www.forbes.com/sites/kionasmith/2017/10/11/whats-in-the-smallpox-vaccine/

137. 2015 Summary Health Statistics, https://ftp.cdc.gov/pub/Health_Statistics/NCHS/NHIS/SHS/2015_SHS_Table_A-2.pdf

138. *http://www.crohnscolitisfoundation.org/what-are-crohns-and-colitis/what-is-crohns-disease/*

139. Sanderson, J D et al. "Mycobacterium Paratuberculosis DNA in Crohn's Disease Tissue." Gut 33.7 (1992): 890–896. Print.

140. Orr MM, Tamarind DL, Cook J, et al. "Preliminary studies on the response of rabbit bowel to intramural injection of L form bacteria" (abstr). Br J Surg 1974;61:921.

141. Shepherd NA, Crocker PR, Smith AP, Levison DA., "Exogenous pigment in Peyer's patches," Hum Pathol. 1987 Jan;18(1):50-4.

142. Urbanski SJ1, Arsenault AL, Green FH, Haber G., "Pigment resembling atmospheric dust in Peyer's patches," Mod Pathol. 1989 May;2(3):222-6.

143. Pineton de Chambrun, G et al. "Aluminum Enhances Inflammation and Decreases Mucosal Healing in Experimental Colitis in Mice." Mucosal Immunology 7.3 (2014): 589–601. PMC. Web. 2 Jan. 2018.

144. LERNER, A. (2007), Aluminum Is a Potential Environmental Factor for Crohn's Disease Induction. Annals of the New York Academy of Sciences, 1107: 329–345. doi:10.1196/annals.1381.035

145. Perl, Daniel P., Fogarty, Ursula, Harpaz, Noam, Sachar, David B., "Bacterial-Metal Interactions: The Potential Role of Aluminum and Other Trace Elements in the Etiology of Chrohn's Disease," Inflamm Bowel Dis • Volume 10, Number 6, November 2004.

146. Stabel JR1, Lambertz A., "Efficacy of pasteurization conditions for the inactivation of Mycobacterium avium subsp. paratuberculosis in milk," J Food Prot. 2004 Dec;67(12):2719-26.

147. Sartor RB, Rath HC, Sellon RK, et al. (1996) Microbial factors in chronic intestinal inflammation. Curr Opp Gastroenterol 12:327–333.

148. Bamba T, Matsuda H, Endo M, et al. (1995) The pathogenic role of Bacteroides vulgatus in patients with ulcerative colitis. J Gastroenterol 30(8 Suppl):45–47.

149. Gillberg, J. Carina, et. al, "AUTISTIC BEHAVIOUR AND ATTENTION DEFICITS IN TUBEROUS SCLEROSIS: A POPULATION-BASED STUDY", Developmental Medicine & Child Neurology, Vol 36, Issue 1, p. 50-56, http://dx.doi.org/10.1111/j.1469-8749.1994.tb11765.x

150. Gipson, Tanjala T et al. "Potential for Treatment of Severe Autism in Tuberous Sclerosis Complex." World Journal of Clinical Pediatrics 2.3 (2013): 16–25. PMC. Web. 22 Dec. 2017.

151. Jeste, Shafali Spurling, "TSC and Autism Spectrum Disorders", Tuberous Sclerosis Alliance, September 2013, http://www.tsalliance.org/about-tsc/signs-and-symptoms-of-tsc/brain-and-neurological-function/tsc-and-autism-spectrum-disorders/

152. *https://www.inspire.com/groups/tuberous-sclerosis-alliance/discussion/brain-tumors-keep-developing-what-does-that-mean/?ga=freshen*

153. https://www.cdc.gov/media/releases/2016/s0413-zika-microcephaly.html

154. https://www.npr.org/sections/goatsandsoda/2017/03/30/521925733/why-didnt-zika-cause-a-surge-in-microcephaly-in-2016

155. PAVITHRA L. CHAVALI et. al, "Neurodevelopmental protein Musashi-1 interacts with the Zika genome and promotes viral replication", SCIENCE07 JUL 2017 : 83-88

156. LING YUAN et. al, "A single mutation in the prM protein of Zika virus contributes to fetal microcephaly", Published Online Science, Sep. 28, 2017

157. *http://crooked-theory.s3.amazonaws.com/BrazilanHealthOffice-TechnicalMemo-TDaP-Pregnancy-2014.pdf*

158. *Worth, Katie, "As Brazil Confronts Zika, Vaccine Rumors Shape Perceptions," Frontline: PBS, February 16, 2016, https://www.pbs.org/wgbh/frontline/article/as-brazil-confronts-zika-vaccine-rumors-shape-perceptions/*

159. "Former doctor gets probation in Junior Seau case," Schrotenboer, Brent, USA Today, Jan. 5, 2017,

https://www.usatoday.com/story/sports/nfl/2017/01/05/david-chao-chargers-doctor-settlement-junior-seau-death/96226836/

160. *John Haslam, Observations on Madness and Melancholy (London: G. Hayden, 1809), p. 259-260.*

161. *Emil Kraepelin, General Paresis (New York: The Journal of Nervous and Mental Disease, 1913), p. 2.*

162. Ibid., p. 5

163. 26Thomas W. Salmon, "General Paralysis as a Public Health Problem," American Journal of Insanity, 1914, 71: 41– 50.

164. "Health, United States, 2016 with Chartbook on Long-term trends in Health", U.S. Department of Health and Human Services, Table 19

165. McGEER, P. L., ITAGAKI, S., TAGO, H. and McGEER, E. G. (1988), Occurrence of HLA-DR Reactive Microglia in Alzheimer's Disease. Annals of the New York Academy of Sciences, 540: 319–323. doi: 10.1111/j.1749-6632.1988.tb27086.x

166. Joseph Rogers, Scott Webster, Lih-Fen Lue, Libuse Brachova, W. Harold Civin, Mark Emmerling, Brenda Shivers, Douglas Walker, Patrick McGeer, Inflammation and Alzheimer's disease pathogenesis, In Neurobiology of Aging, Volume 17, Issue 5, 1996, Pages 681-686, ISSN 0197-4580, https://doi.org/10.1016/0197-4580(96)00115-7.

167. Perry, V. Hugh, Cunningham, Colm, Holmes, Clive, Systemic infections and inflammation affect chronic neurodegeneration, Nature Reviews Immunology, January 15, 2007, Vol. 7, 161, http://dx.doi.org/10.1038/nri2015

168. Corinna Van Den Heuvel, Emma Thornton, Robert Vink, Traumatic brain injury and Alzheimer's disease: a review, Editor(s): John T. Weber, Andrew I.R. Maas, In Progress in Brain Research, Elsevier, Volume 161, 2007, Pages 303-316, https://doi.org/10.1016/S0079-6123(06)61021-2

169. https://www.alz.org/alzheimers_disease_myths_about_alzheimers.asp

170. Mirza A , King A , Troakes C , Exley C ((2017)) Aluminium in brain tissue in familial Alzheimer's disease. J Trace Elem Med Biol 40: , 30–36.

171. Oshima E , Ishihara T , Yokota O , Nakashima-Yasuda H , Nagao S , Ikeda C , Naohara J , Terada S , Uchitomi Y ((2013)) Accelerated tau aggregation, apoptosis and neurological dysfunction caused by chronic oral administration of aluminum in a mouse model of tauopathies. Brain Pathol 23: , 633–644.

172. Yan, D., Jin, C., Cao, Y., Wang, L., Lu, X., Yang, J., Wu, S. and Cai, Y. (2017), Effects of Aluminium on Long-Term Memory in Rats and on SIRT1 Mediating the Transcription of CREB-Dependent Gene in Hippocampus. Basic Clin Pharmacol Toxicol, 121: 342–352. doi:10.1111/bcpt.12798

173. Edwardson JA , Moore PB , Ferrier IN , Lilley JS , Newton GWA , Barker J , Templar J , Day JP ((1993)) Effect of silicon on gastrointestinal absorption of aluminium. Lancet 342: , 211–212.

174. Moore PB , Edwardson JA , Ferrier IN , Taylor GA , Tyrer SP , Day JP , King SJ , Lilley JS ((1997)) Gastrointestinal absorption of aluminum is increased in Down's syndrome. Biol Psychiatry 41: , 488–492.

175. Maheshwari, Priya | Eslick, Guy D., "Bacterial Infection and Alzheimer's Disease: A Meta-Analysis," J Alzheimers Dis. 2015;43(3):957-66. doi: 10.3233/JAD-140621.

176. MacIntyre, A., Abramov, R., Hammond, C.J., Hudson, A.P., Arking, E.J., Little, C.S., Appelt, D.M. and Balin, B.J. (2003), Chlamydia pneumoniae infection promotes the transmigration of monocytes through human brain endothelial cells. J. Neurosci. Res., 71: 740–750. doi:10.1002/jnr.10519

177. Exley, Christopher, "Aluminum Should Now Be Considered a Primary Etiological Factor in Alzheimer's Disease," Journal of Alzheimer's Disease Reports, vol. 1, no. 1, pp. 23-25, 2017, https://doi.org/10.3233/ADR-170010

178. Ibid.

179. Jones, David A. "Changes in the Force–velocity Relationship of Fatigued Muscle: Implications for Power Production and Possible Causes." The Journal of Physiology 588.Pt 16 (2010): 2977–2986. PMC. Web. 4 Jan. 2018.

180. Tucker, R., Rauch, L., Harley, Y.X. et al. Pflugers Arch - Eur J Physiol (2004) 448: 422. https://doi.org/10.1007/s00424-004-1267-4

181. Sloniger MA1, Cureton KJ, Prior BM, Evans EM., "Anaerobic capacity and muscle activation during horizontal and uphill running," J Appl Physiol (1985). 1997 Jul;83(1):262-9.

182. Guimarães, J. B., Wanner, S. P., Machado, S. C., Lima, M. R. M., Cordeiro, L. M. S., Pires, W., La Guardia, R. B., Silami-Garcia, E., Rodrigues, L. O. C. and Lima, N. R. V. (2013), Fatigue is mediated by cholinoceptors within the ventromedial hypothalamus independent of changes in core temperature. Scandinavian Journal of Medicine & Science in Sports, 23: 46–56.

183. *Gibson H, Carroll N, Clague JE, Edwards RH. Exercise performance and fatiguability in patients with chronic fatigue syndrome. J Neurol Neurosurg Psychiatry 1993; 56: 993±8.*

184. Russell D. Romeo, Rudy Bellani, Ilia N. Karatsoreos, Nara Chhua, Mary Vernov, Cheryl D. Conrad, Bruce S. McEwen; Stress History and Pubertal Development Interact to Shape Hypothalamic-Pituitary-Adrenal Axis Plasticity, Endocrinology, Volume 147, Issue 4, 1 April 2006, Pages 1664–1674, https://doi.org/10.1210/en.2005-1432.

185. L. Ian Schmitt, Ralf D. Wimmer, Miho Nakajima, Michael Happ, Sima Mofakham & Michael M. Halass, "Thalamic amplification of cortical connectivity sustains attentional control," Nature 545, 219–223 (11 May 2017), doi:10.1038/nature22073.

186. Ab Aziz, Che Badariah, and Asma Hayati Ahmad. "The Role of the Thalamus in Modulating Pain." The Malaysian Journal of Medical Sciences: MJMS 13.2 (2006): 11–18. Print.

187. *https://www.webmd.com/rheumatoid-arthritis/understanding-juvenile-rheumatoid-arthritis-basics#1*

188. Li S, Yu Y, Yue Y, Zhang Z, Su K. Microbial Infection and Rheumatoid Arthritis. Journal of clinical & cellular immunology. 2013;4(6):174. doi:10.4172/2155-9899.1000174.

189. Nuutti Vartiainen, Caroline Perchet, Michel Magnin, Christelle Creac'h, Philippe Convers, Norbert Nighoghossian, François Mauguière, Roland Peyron, Luis Garcia-Larrea; Thalamic pain: anatomical and physiological indices of prediction, Brain, Volume 139, Issue 3, 1 March 2016, Pages 708–722, https://doi.org/10.1093/brain/awv389.

190. M. Steriade and R. R. Llinás, "The functional states of the thalamus and the associated neuronal interplay," Physiological Reviews 1988 68:3, 649-742.

191. Mikael Knip, Riitta Veijola, Suvi M. Virtanen, Heikki Hyöty, Outi Vaarala, Hans K. Åkerblom, "Environmental Triggers and Determinants of Type 1 Diabetes," Diabetes Dec 2005, 54 (suppl 2) S125-S136; DOI: 10.2337/diabetes.54.suppl_2.S125

192. Nam, Sung Min et al. "Reduction of Adult Hippocampal Neurogenesis Is Amplified by Aluminum Exposure in a Model of Type 2 Diabetes." Journal of Veterinary Science 17.1 (2016): 13–20. PMC. Web. 28 Dec. 2017.

193. M C Honeyman, B S Coulson, N L Stone, S A Gellert, P N Goldwater, C E Steele, J J Couper, B D Tait, P G Colman, L C Harrison, "Association between rotavirus infection and pancreatic islet autoimmunity in children at risk of developing type 1 diabetes," Diabetes Aug 2000, 49 (8) 1319-1324; DOI: 10.2337/diabetes.49.8.1319

194. Capua, Ilaria et al. "Influenza A Viruses Grow in Human Pancreatic Cells and Cause Pancreatitis and Diabetes in an Animal Model." Journal of Virology 87.1 (2013): 597–610. PMC. Web. 28 Dec. 2017.

195. Chen, Cheng et al. "Cadmium Exposure and Risk of Pancreatic Cancer: A Meta-Analysis of Prospective Cohort Studies and Case-Control Studies among Individuals without Occupational Exposure History." Environmental science and pollution research international 22.22 (2015): 17465–17474. PMC. Web. 28 Dec. 2017.

196. *Ionescu-Tîrgoviste, Constantin. Etienne Lancereaux (1829-1910) [internet]. 2014 Aug 13; Diapedia 1104337136 rev. no. 8. Available from: https://doi.org/10.14496/dia.1104337136.8*

197. Johan Askling, Johan Grunewald, Anders Eklund, Gunnar Hillerdal, and Anders Ekbom, "Increased Risk for Cancer Following Sarcoidosis," https://doi.org/10.1164/ajrccm.160.5.9904045   PubMed: 10556138.

198. Ishige I1, Eishi Y, Takemura T, Kobayashi I, Nakata K, Tanaka I, Nagaoka S, Iwai K, Watanabe K, Takizawa T, Koike M., "Propionibacterium acnes is the most common bacterium commensal in peripheral lung tissue and mediastinal lymph nodes from subjects without sarcoidosis," Sarcoidosis Vasc Diffuse Lung Dis. 2005 Mar;22(1):33-42.

199. Winters, Ryan, Masatoshi Kida, and Kumarasen Cooper. "Hamazaki-Wesenberg Bodies in Two Patients with No History of Sarcoidosis." Journal of Clinical Pathology 60.10 (2007): 1169–1171. PMC.

200. John H. Lee, James H. O'Keefe, David Bell, Donald D. Hensrud, Michael F. Holick, Vitamin D Deficiency: An Important, Common, and Easily Treatable Cardiovascular Risk Factor?, In Journal of the American College of Cardiology, Volume 52, Issue 24, 2008, Pages 1949-1956, ISSN 0735-1097, https://doi.org/10.1016/j.jacc.2008.08.050.

201. Y. Oren, Y. Shapira, N. Agmon-Levin, S. Kivity, Y. Zafrir, A. Altman, A. Lerner and Y. Shoenfeld, "Vitamin D insufficiency in a sunny environment: a demographic and seasonal analysis," Isr Med Assoc J. 2010 Dec;12(12):751-6.

202. Fairweather D, Frisancho-Kiss S, Rose NR. Sex Differences in Autoimmune Disease from a

Pathological Perspective. The American Journal of Pathology. 2008;173(3):600-609. doi:10.2353/ajpath. 2008.071008.

203. Viganò P1, Lattuada D, Mangioni S, Ermellino L, Vignali M, Caporizzo E, Panina-Bordignon P, Besozzi M, Di Blasio AM., "Cycling and early pregnant endometrium as a site of regulated expression of the vitamin D system," J Mol Endocrinol. 2006 Jun;36(3):415-24.

204. Proal, A. D., Albert, P. J. and Marshall, T. G. (2009), Dysregulation of the Vitamin D Nuclear Receptor May Contribute to the Higher Prevalence of Some Autoimmune Diseases in Women. Annals of the New York Academy of Sciences, 1173: 252–259. doi:10.1111/j.1749-6632.2009.04672.x.

205. Bennett RG, Heimann DG, Tuma DJ. Relaxin Reduces Fibrosis in Models of Progressive and Established Hepatic Fibrosis. Annals of the New York Academy of Sciences. 2009;1160:348-349. doi: 10.1111/j.1749-6632.2008.03783.x.

206. VanDuyn, Natalia et al. "THE METAL TRANSPORTER SMF-3/DMT-1 MEDIATES ALUMINUM-INDUCED DOPAMINE NEURON DEGENERATION." Journal of neurochemistry 124.1 (2013): 147–157. PMC. Web. 30 Dec. 2017.

207. Hasna Erazi, Samir Ahboucha, Halima Gamrani, "Chronic exposure to aluminum reduces tyrosine hydroxylase expression in the substantia nigra and locomotor performance in rats," Neuroscience Letters, Volume 487, Issue 1, 2011, Pages 8-11, ISSN 0304-3940, https://doi.org/10.1016/j.neulet.2010.09.053.

208. Wenk GL, Stemmer KL., "The influence of ingested aluminum upon norepinephrine and dopamine levels in the rat brain," Neurotoxicology. 1981 Oct;2(2):347-53.

209. Paul F. Good, C.W. Olanow, Daniel P. Perl, Neuromelanin-containing neurons of the substantia nigra accumulate iron and aluminum in Parkinson's disease: a LAMMA study, In Brain Research, Volume 593, Issue 2, 1992, Pages 343-346, ISSN 0006-8993, https://doi.org/10.1016/0006-8993(92)91334-B.

210. Makoto Sasaki; Eri Shibata; Koujiro Tohyama; Junko Takahashi; Kotaro Otsuka; Kuniaki Tsuchiya; Satoshi Takahashi; Shigeru Ehara; Yasuo Terayama; Akio Sakai, "Neuromelanin magnetic resonance imaging of locus ceruleus and substantia nigra in Parkinson's disease," NeuroReport. 17(11):1215-1218, JUL 2006, DOI: 10.1097/01.wnr.0000227984.84927.a7 , PMID: 16837857.

211. Meglio L1, Oteiza PI, "Aluminum enhances melanin-induced lipid peroxidation," Neurochem Res. 1999 Aug;24(8):1001-8.

212. B. Mirza, H. Hadberg, P. Thomsen, and T. Moos, "The absence of reactive astrocytosis is indicative of a unique inflammatory process in Parkinson's disease," Neuroscience, vol. 95, no. 2, pp. 425–432, 1999.

213. Zhang W, Zecca L, Wilson B, et al. Human neuromelanin: an endogenous microglial activator for dopaminergic neuron death. Frontiers in bioscience (Elite edition). 2013;5:1-11.

214. "Progressive Supranuclear Palsy Fact Sheet," National Institute of Neurological Disorders and Stroke, https://www.ninds.nih.gov/Disorders/Patient-Caregiver-Education/Fact-Sheets/Progressive-Supranuclear-Palsy-Fact-Sheet

215. Watad A, David P, Brown S, Shoenfeld Y. Autoimmune/Inflammatory Syndrome Induced by Adjuvants and Thyroid Autoimmunity. Frontiers in Endocrinology. 2016;7:150. doi:10.3389/fendo. 2016.00150.

216. George J. Kahaly, Martin P. Hansen, Type 1 diabetes associated autoimmunity, In Autoimmunity Reviews, Volume 15, Issue 7, 2016, Pages 644-648, ISSN 1568-9972, https://doi.org/10.1016/j.autrev. 2016.02.017.

217. Kim D., "Low vitamin D status is associated with hypothyroid Hashimoto's thyroiditis," Hormones (Athens). 2016 Jul;15(3):385-393. doi: 10.14310/horm.2002.1681.

218. Xiaofei Wang, Wenli Cheng, Yu Ma & Jingqiang Zhu, "Vitamin D receptor gene FokI but not TaqI, ApaI, BsmI polymorphism is associated with Hashimoto's thyroiditis: a meta-analysis," Scientific Reports 7, Article number: 41540 (2017), doi:10.1038/srep41540.

219. Page, C., Duverlie, G., Sevestre, H. and Desailloud, R. (2015), Erythrovirus B19 and autoimmune thyroid diseases. Review of the literature and pathophysiological hypotheses. J. Med. Virol., 87: 162–169. doi:10.1002/jmv.23963.

220. Burfeind KG, Yadav V, Marks DL. Hypothalamic Dysfunction and Multiple Sclerosis: Implications for Fatigue and Weight Dysregulation. Current neurology and neuroscience reports. 2016;16(11):98. doi: 10.1007/s11910-016-0700-3.

221. Sandra V. Verstraeten, Mari S. Golub, Carl L. Keen, Patricia I. Oteiza, "Myelin Is a Preferential Target of Aluminum-Mediated Oxidative Damage, In Archives of Biochemistry and Biophysics," Volume 344,

Issue 2, 1997, Pages 289-294, ISSN 0003-9861, https://doi.org/10.1006/abbi.1997.0146.

222. Fulgenzi A, Vietti D, Ferrero ME. Aluminium Involvement in Neurotoxicity. BioMed Research International. 2014;2014:758323. doi:10.1155/2014/758323.

223. Fulgenzi, A., Zanella, S.G., Mariani, M.M. et al., "A case of multiple sclerosis improvement following removal of heavy metal intoxication," Biometals (2012) 25: 569. https://doi.org/10.1007/s10534-012-9537-7.

224. Dal Bianco, A., Bradl, M., Frischer, J., Kutzelnigg, A., Jellinger, K. and Lassmann, H. (2008), "Multiple sclerosis and Alzheimer's disease," Ann Neurol., 63: 174–183. doi:10.1002/ana.21240

225. Hilton DA, Love S, Fletcher A, Pringle JH., "Absence of Epstein-Barr virus RNA in multiple sclerosis as assessed by in situ hybridisation," Journal of Neurology, Neurosurgery, and Psychiatry. 1994;57(8): 975-976.

226. Chatzipanagiotou, S., Tsakanikas, C., Anagnostouli, M. et al., "Detection of Chlamydia Pneumoniae in the Cerebrospinal Fluid of Patients with Multiple Sclerosis by Combination of Cell Culture and PCR," CNS Drugs (2003) 7: 41. https://doi.org/10.1007/BF03260019.

227. Moses H Jr1, Sriram S., "An infectious basis for multiple sclerosis: perspectives on the role of Chlamydia pneumoniae and other agents," BioDrugs. 2001;15(3):199-206.

228. Alharbi FM. Update in vitamin D and multiple sclerosis. Neurosciences. 2015;20(4):329-335. doi: 10.17712/nsj.2015.4.20150357.

229. Bulkley, L. Duncan, "Eczema With an Analysis of Eight Thousand Cases of the Disease," G.P.Putnam's Sons: London, 1901.

230. Kuitunen M1, "Probiotics and prebiotics in preventing food allergy and eczema," Curr Opin Allergy Clin Immunol. 2013 Jun;13(3):280-6. doi: 10.1097/ACI.0b013e328360ed66.

231. Nylund L, Nermes M, Isolauri E, Salminen S, de Vos WM, Satokari R. Severity of atopic disease inversely correlates with intestinal microbiota diversity and butyrate-producing bacteria. Allergy 2015; 70: 241–244.

232. Ferritin as an indicator of suspected iron deficiency in children with autism spectrum disorder: prevalence of low serum ferritin concentration.
Dosman CF, et al Dev Med Child Neurol. 2006 Dec;48(12):1008-9

233. Iron deficiency in autism and Asperger syndrome.
Latif A, Heinz P, Cook R. Autism. 2002 Mar;6(1):103-14.

234. Konofal E, Lecendreux M, Arnulf I, Mouren M. Iron Deficiency in Children With Attention-Deficit/Hyperactivity Disorder. Arch Pediatr Adolesc Med. 2004;158(12):1113–1115. doi:10.1001/archpedi.158.12.1113.

235. Kaiser, Lana et al., "Aluminum-Induced Anemia," American Journal of Kidney Diseases , Volume 6, Issue 5, 348-352.

236. Simone A Nouér, Marcio Nucci & Elias Anaissie, "Tackling antibiotic resistance in febrile neutropenia: current challenges with and recommendations for managing infections with resistant Gram-negative organisms," Expert Review of Hematology Vol. 8, Iss. 5, 2015.

237. Ngeh J, Gupta S, Goodbourn C, Panayiotou B, McElligott G, "Chlamydia pneumoniae in Elderly Patients with Stroke (C-PEPS): A Case-Control Study on the Seroprevalence of Chlamydia pneumoniae in Elderly Patients with Acute Cerebrovascular Disease," Cerebrovasc Dis 2003;15:11-16

238. IZADI, Morteza et al. Chlamydia pneumoniae in the atherosclerotic plaques of coronary artery disease patients.. Acta Medica Iranica, [S.l.], p. 864-870, Dec. 2013. ISSN 1735-9694.

239. Shrikhande Sunanda N, Zodpey Sanjay P, Negandhi Himanshu, "A case-control study examining association between infectious agents and acute myocardial infarction," Indian J Public Health. 2014 Apr-Jun;58(2):106-9. doi: 10.4103/0019-557X.132285.

240. Kytö V, Sipilä J, Rautava P The effects of gender and age on occurrence of clinically suspected myocarditis in adulthood Heart 2013;99:1681-1684.

241. http://www.childrenshospital.org/conditions-and-treatments/conditions/torticollis

242. *Bell, Sir Charles, "The nervous system of the human body : embracing the papers delivered to the Royal Society on the subject of the nerves" (Washington : Stereotyped by D. Green, for the Register and Library of Medical and Chirurgical Science, 1833), p. 166-167.*

243. *Olmsted, Dan; Blaxill, Mark. The Age of Autism: Mercury, Medicine, and a Man-Made Epidemic (Kindle Locations 6415-6418). St. Martin's Press. Kindle Edition.*

Other popular books by **Forrest Maready:**

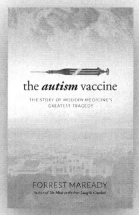

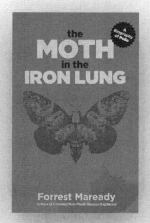

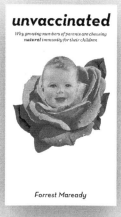

The Autism Vaccine:
The story of modern medicine's greatest tragedy

The Moth in the Iron Lung:
A Biography of Polio

Unvaccinated:
Why growing numbers of parents are choosing natural immunity for their children

Available at select retailers and:

www.**forrestmaready**.com

Made in the USA
Monee, IL
04 December 2021

83853594R00229